Practice Development Workbook for Nursing, Health and Social Care Teams

Professor Jan Dewing
Head of Person-centred Research and Practice Development, East Sussex Healthcare NHS Trust, Eastbourne, UK
Co-Director, Centre for Practice Development (including Lead for Kent Sussex Surrey, Dementia Care Innovation Hub), Canterbury Christchurch University, Canterbury, UK
Visiting Professor, Person-centred Practice Research Centre, University of Ulster, Ulster, Northern Ireland
Visiting Professor, School of Nursing & Midwifery University of Wollongong, Wollongong NSW, Australia

Professor Brendan McCormack
Director, Institute of Nursing and Health Research and Head of the Person-centred Practice Research Centre, University of Ulster, Ulster, Northern Ireland
Professor II, Buskerud University College, Drammen, Norway
Adjunct Professor of Nursing, University of Technology, Sydney, Australia
Visiting Professor, School of Medicine & Dentistry, University of Aberdeen, Aberdeen, Scotland

Professor Angie Titchen
Independent Practice Development Consultant
Principal Investigator, Knowledge Centre for Evidence-Based Practice, Fontys University of Applied Sciences, Eindhoven, The Netherlands
Visiting Professor, University of Ulster, Ulster, Northern Ireland
Adjunct Professor, Charles Sturt University, Bathurst NSW, Australia
Associate Fellow, University of Warwick, Warwick, UK

WILEY Blackwell

This edition first published 2014 © 2014 by John Wiley & Sons, Ltd

Registered office: John Wiley & Sons, Ltd, The Atrium, Southern Gate, Chichester, West Sussex, PO19 8SQ, UK

Editorial offices: 9600 Garsington Road, Oxford, OX4 2DQ, UK
The Atrium, Southern Gate, Chichester, West Sussex, PO19 8SQ, UK
111 River Street, Hoboken, NJ 07030-5774, USA

For details of our global editorial offices, for customer services and for information about how to apply for permission to reuse the copyright material in this book please see our website at www.wiley.com/wiley-blackwell

The right of the author to be identified as the author of this work has been asserted in accordance with the UK Copyright, Designs and Patents Act 1988.

Library of Congress Cataloging-in-Publication Data
Dewing, Jan, author.
  Practice development workbook for nursing, health and social care teams / Jan Dewing, Brendan McCormack, Angie Titchen.
    1 online resource.
  Includes bibliographical references and index.
  Description based on print version record and CIP data provided by publisher; resource not viewed.
  ISBN 978-1-118-67649-3 (Adobe PDF) – ISBN 978-1-118-67675-2 (ePub) – ISBN 978-1-118-67670-7 (pbk.)
  I. McCormack, Brendan, author.   II. Titchen, Angie, author.   III. Title.
  [DNLM: 1. Patient-Centered Care–organization & administration.   2. Delivery of Health Care, Integrated–organization & administration.   3. Professional Practice–organization & administration.   4. Staff Development–methods.   W 84.7]
  RT90.5
  610.73068–dc 3

                              2014006442

A catalogue record for this book is available from the British Library.

Wiley also publishes its books in a variety of electronic formats. Some content that appears in print may not be available in electronic books.

Cover image: iStock © Mr-Spilberg
Cover design by Meaden Creative

Set in 9/12.5 pt FrutigerLTStd-Cn by Toppan Best-set Premedia Limited
Printed and bound by CPI Group (UK) Ltd, Croydon, CR0 4YY

C9781118676707_061224

Table of contents

Preface

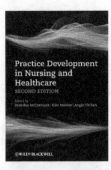

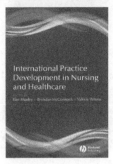

This workbook can be used on its own or to support *Practice Development in Nursing and Healthcare* (McCormack et al., 2013) and *International Practice Development in Nursing and Healthcare* (Manley et al., 2009). These two books make an important contribution to understanding practice development and its purposes in contemporary health and social care. This new workbook takes practice developers and others involved in practice development through each step of a typical practice development journey. This practical text offers readers the opportunity to learn how to carry out key practice development methods and activities in the workplace with colleagues, service users and others.

Practice Development Workbook for Nursing, Health and Social Care Teams explores a wide range of practice development methods, tools and processes to help those engaging in practice development to become more skilled and confident at taking part in or facilitating and leading practice development activity in a variety of health and social care contexts.

The workbook aims to enable readers to be confident in their approaches to practice development and bringing about sustainable culture change that involves service users and staff throughout the organisation. The time is right for this book. Internationally, it is increasingly recognised that an effective culture is central to patients receiving the highest quality care and health care staff being able to provide it. The need to have workplace cultures that enable staff to do the best they can, that the conditions for staff to be able to have critically reflective conversations and that help service users and staff to engage effectively is a priority agenda in health systems.

This book is aimed therefore at health and social care practitioners in a variety of roles, such as clinical practice, education, research and quality improvement managers, patient-safety and service improvement facilitators and students, as well as those with a primary practice development role and across health and social care sectors.

About the companion website

Please also visit the companion website:
www.wiley.com/go/practicedevelopment/workbook
The website includes valuable material for you to print out and use:

- Evaluation tools
- Questionnaires and checklists
- Worksheets and reflection tools
- Sample presentations in PowerPoint format
- A bonus online chapter on sharing and celebrating

The website material supplements, and is organised around, the chapters in the workbook.

Chapter 1 Introduction: Getting the Best Out of This Resource

Contents

Introduction

> *I thought that we knew best what was good for the people here. Now I know that we don't and even if we do, it's not always what the person wants. Practice Development has shown me that what I know is important but how I talk to and value what people want and do not want is more important (Care worker's reflection). (McCormack et al., 2010)*

This resource is firmly based in care practice and uses a person-centred practice development approach. It is relevant to all health and social care professionals across a multitude of settings. By paying attention to developing person-centred cultures in care settings (hospital and community based) and care homes, the conditions to 'grow' person-centredness for patients, service users and residents can be created. These conditions of course need a learning culture within the workplace and the organisation or care home to thrive. A learning culture helps care teams to be reflective about their work, to learn in and from work and to evaluate their effectiveness. This culture also supports teams, their leaders and managers in developing helping or facilitation skills across the team. Look at these examples from East Sussex Healthcare NHS Trust on the south coast of England.

> *Inspired by a practice development session at their hospital, Lizzie and Katherine asked their local practice development lead for support with finding out what patients really thought of their care and of their experiences. Lizzie and Katherine started with just an idea about what they would like to do although they didn't know how to collect their evidence. After a few informal discussion sessions they had a plan for what they would do (patient stories), why and how. They commented that the barriers they thought would deter them no longer seemed such a problem.*
>
> *A therapist working in a rehabilitation unit, and developing her facilitation skills, learned how to do this by committing to clinical supervision and becoming a supervisor for other practitioners. Within a year she was leading action learning sets in the unit and could identify how she was using her facilitation skills in many other aspects of her role.*

Also, see what team members say who have experienced developing their practice in a care home in the way we are offering you in this resource (adapted from McCormack et al., 2010).

> *Mary identified the lack of Catering involvement with the people who live in their homes other than through the provision of food. For example, many in the catering department could not identify people*

---

who live in the home by their face. This brought about the 'Face to the Plate' development where a photo of each person who lives in the home was placed on their menu sheet.

Mary describes the processes she used: I spoke to staff about this and I asked them to introduce the catering staff to people who live in the homes so that residents could tell the catering staff a little about themselves. I further developed this new relationship by talking with the catering manager. We explored other ways to involve the catering team with people who live in the home's care. Now they take part in social activities such as outings and sitting down with a cup of tea in the dining room at breakfast time to talk with people who live in the homes. They will also be involved in helping the selection of daily menu choices within the coming weeks, and some are now part of our person-centred working group. (Registered Nurse)

We have been overly obsessed by tasks in my team. I am developing a greater awareness of how this gets in the way of being person-centred. However, it is only when we all have a similar awareness that we become truly person-centred in the way we work. How I achieve this whilst working in a busy community team is my challenge! (Therapy assistant)

Team members started the day by reviewing how they would schedule the different activities that needed to be done with patients and identified who needed to be involved. The plan included those activities (such as showering) that could be undertaken in the afternoon as a more 'relaxing activity' as opposed to a 'morning task' . . . it was good to see team members check with each other what help they needed with their work.

Welcome to this *Practice Development Workbook for Nursing, Health and Social Care Teams*. Developed by a team with expertise in practice development, from the England Centre for Practice Development at the Canterbury Christchurch University and the University of Ulster, these resources can help you and your colleagues to improve the care you offer patients/clients and other service users (or residents) and families in your service(s). We believe these resources will be particularly useful to experienced and new or novice practice developers because of the way we have designed them to be used and the options and guidance we offer throughout. Whilst the focus of this resource is to enable the provision of enhanced or better care for patients and residents, its use could help you and others have a much wider impact in your service/care home or across your organisation. This could include you feeling more knowledgeable and confident, the development of more person-centred relationships with patients/ residents and families, more power sharing and joint decision-making between service or care home managers and team members and developing a culture that enables everyone there to feel valued, respected and helped to achieve their full potential.

Although we refer to this as a 'resource' it can also form a workbook for individuals or small groups of practitioners to work through in their workplaces or as part of a programme or academic module. Many of the resources, learning activities and tools in this resource have been developed, tested, revised and collected, over several years, by the authors in collaboration with other practitioners with whom they have worked in a variety of settings, including hospital, community, residential and nursing care homes. In a few cases there are resources developed by other practice developers and practitioners in associated fields (such as education and research). As far as possible, original sources are acknowledged and references provided.

You will note that a few of the resources offered are specific to engaging patients and residents with dementia in practice development. They are here for two reasons. The first relates to evidence that the number of older people being cared for in health and social care settings is growing significantly. Whatever setting or profession you are in, you are increasingly likely to be working with patients/residents with dementia at some point. The second reason concerns the assumption that patients/residents with dementia or severe cognitive impairment cannot meaningfully engage in practice development (or research or evaluation for that matter) nor can they give consent. So they tend to be excluded.

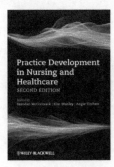

However, over the last few years, great strides have been made in developing approaches to include patients/residents with dementia and severe cognitive impairment in practice development and research. Some of these approaches are therefore offered here with practical guidance to help care staff include such patients/residents in practice development work.

Finally, this workbook can be used alongside the material on the companion website (**www.wiley.com/go/ practicedevelopment/workbook**) and the book *Practice Development in Nursing and Healthcare* (McCormack et al., 2013). This more theoretical book contains up-to-date thinking on practice development that is illustrated with real-life examples. This workbook is the perfect partner as it provides tools, learning materials and practical know-how about how to put this thinking into action.

Aim of the resource

The purpose of bringing together this resource is to:

> offer practical guidance, practice development learning activities and tools that can be used by teams (and patients/residents and families) in care settings within the work place and working day to make changes to the way care is planned and delivered and ultimately to make a positive difference to the lives of service users and those who work with them.

We see the resource as providing you and your colleagues with a comprehensive collection and choice of materials and learning activities that will enable you to move closer towards offering person-centred care and services. We aim to make this collection user-friendly by including material that has already been tested for use in health and social care settings and thus in 'real-life' situations by teams. As you engage with the materials and activities, you will be learning about the range of skills for becoming more person-centred and at the same time contributing to developing the culture that is needed to support and sustain person-centredness in your workplace.

This resource matters because . . .

Compliance, quality improvement and innovation are all part of our work. You will be probably only too aware of inspection and regulation requirements across health and social care services. Adopting an approach to continuous practice development that ensures that you are continuously developing your practice will really help with meeting these standards. In all its strategy work, the Department of Health and similar bodies in other countries has shown that it values the efforts made to ensure high quality care for people. However, it also recognises that we all need help to continuously develop and do our best. This resource can help teams learn more about how to give the kind of care they would like to give, given the chance.

Compliance

By law, all health and social care services are responsible for making sure that the care and treatment they provide meet government standards of quality and safety. In England for example, the Care Quality Commission (CQC) registers services if they can show that they are meeting government standards. The CQC inspects services to assess that they continue to meet the government standards and will take different levels of action if they don't. Similarly, care at home or in care homes (at the GPs or at a dentist) is also regulated and inspected by the CQC.

The five standards for health and social care (aimed at service users) are as follows.

1. You should expect to be respected, involved in your care and support, and told what's happening at every stage.
2. You should expect care, treatment and support that meets your needs.
3. You should expect to be safe.
4. You should expect to be cared for by staff with the right skills to do their jobs properly.
5. You should expect your care provider to routinely check the quality of their services.

(www.cqc.org.uk/public/what-are-standards/government-standards)

Quality

There are many indicators and standards for quality within health and social care. Here we are touching on one framework that puts the patient or service user at the centre. In October 2011 the NHS National Quality Board (NQB) agreed on a working definition of patient experience to guide the measurement of patient experience across the NHS. So was born the NHS Patient Experience Framework, which was launched in 2012, based on a similar framework from the Picker Institute. This framework outlines those elements that are critical to the patients' experience of NHS Services.

- *Respect for patient-centred values, preferences, and expressed needs*, including: cultural issues; the dignity, privacy and independence of patients and service users; an awareness of quality-of-life issues; and shared decision-making.
- *Coordination and integration of care* across the health and social care system.
- *Information, communication, and education* on clinical status, progress, prognosis, and processes of care in order to facilitate autonomy, self-care and health promotion.
- *Physical comfort* including pain management, help with activities of daily living, and clean and comfortable surroundings.
- *Emotional support* and alleviation of fear and anxiety about such issues as clinical status, prognosis, and the impact of illness on patients, their families and their finances.
- *Welcoming the involvement of family and friends*, on whom patients and service users rely, in decision-making and demonstrating awareness and accommodation of their needs as caregivers.
- *Transition and continuity* as regards information that will help patients care for themselves away from a clinical setting, and coordination, planning, and support to ease transitions.
- *Access to care* with attention for example, to time spent waiting for admission or time between admission and placement in a room in an in-patient setting, and waiting time for an appointment or visit in the out-patient, primary care or social care setting.

(www.dh.gov.uk/prod_consum_dh/groups/dh_digitalassets/
@dh/@en/documents/digitalasset/dh_132788.pdf)

Professionally, all registered health and social care practitioners must work within the spirit and the law regarding practice and professional standards. So, you and the way you and your team go about caring for people matters. Most of us would probably say that we are doing the very best we can for patients/residents within the limits placed on us by the busyness and the demanding nature of the work. However, we also know that it is always possible to make further improvements and find creative ways of working with people that lead to better care outcomes.

Who is it for?

This resource is primarily for all health and social care practitioners, service managers in primary, secondary and tertiary care, as well as patients/residents, their families and volunteers, who want, by working together, to improve and develop the way care is given in their care setting or care home. It is for people who want to constantly strive to improve care processes and outcomes. Educators, trainers and project facilitators who go into different care settings might also find this resource useful.

With such a wide array of people involved in health and social care, the resource attempts to offer something for everyone in language that they can understand. As with most new ideas or resources it will take you a little while to become familiar with this resource and everything in it. It is meant to offer a wide range of ideas and materials; there will be some contents that you will find easier to grasp than others and some you will really need to think about before using. And then there will be some materials you will not use. This is the nature of a resource as comprehensive as this one.

> *For me, person-centred care has been in the main about the staff. About developing them to deliver care to people . . . that is of the best quality possible. It's about them learning about their own values and beliefs in order to be able to realise that patients/residents also have a set of values and beliefs that need to be met.*
>
> *My role of facilitator has been in facilitating the growth of the team . . . and supporting them to provide person-centred care. I am very glad I had the opportunity to participate in this programme albeit that on occasion it broke my heart. All I have learned and the networking I have been able to avail of have been of tremendous benefit to me and will continue to be used . . .(Reflection by a Nurse) (Adapted from McCormack et al., 2010)*

Why use this resource?

The resource has the following benefits.

- Using the resource helps you to become more person-centred in your work with patients/residents and colleagues.
- It takes you systematically through the steps of developing practice that many experience as a journey.
- Many of the activities and tools have already been used in health and social care settings and will help teams learn and act alongside the people for whom they care.
- It brings different methods 'alive' and helps you to work with them in practical ways.
- The resource can be used very flexibly within your own workplace by individuals and small groups.
- It will help you to learn, in your workplace, more about your workplace and work and how to improve what you can offer patients/residents and families. This happens through learning spaces rather than training spaces.
- As learning is integrated with developing the way you work, the two happen together. Activities therefore help you to learn at the same time as you are changing things about how you work.
- It will maximise opportunities for all team members to enhance their leadership capability.
- Staff, patients and residents will be actively engaged in designing and collecting data/evidence in the care setting.
- It will help your workplace develop formalised action plans based on priorities in your workplace decided by care staff, patients/residents, families and other stakeholders.
- Patients, residents and their families will be active participants in developing practice.
- Methods of developing the workplace culture will be integrated into everyday care processes, and reflective and development processes.

On first inspection though, it is possible that you might have some very legitimate concerns such as:

> 'Some team members I work with and my managers won't want to use this resource'
> 'I'm not sure it fits with what I do'
> 'It could be misunderstood and misused'
> 'It's too wordy in parts and it has terminology that doesn't mean anything to me'
> 'Knowing how to use it is still an issue especially if there is no one else in the workplace who has the necessary skills to help us'

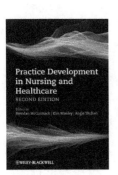

We have been sensitive to these concerns in putting together this resource. We know that practice development including developing workplace culture is an area that perhaps not many people working in health and social care settings know about yet, so we have tried to make the resource as attractive and accessible as possible. We want people to use it! Making it accessible in words that everyone can understand has not been easy due to the diversity of needs in care settings. So, as we say above, we have developed specific parts of this resource for different team members.

Like every area of our work, practice development has its own terminology. When we come new to something, this language can feel to us like jargon. We have tried to make the resources accessible through using as little 'jargon' as possible. We have explained any terminology that might not mean anything to you or that could be misunderstood. We have explained some of the more difficult ideas and principles in materials targeted at staff with professional and vocational qualifications so they will be able explain them to others. We have also tried to be concise, whilst giving you enough detail so that you can engage with or facilitate the activities.

To help you further, we will periodically refer to the book we mentioned earlier: *Practice Development in Nursing and Healthcare* (McCormack et al., 2013). As we said there, this book can help you develop your knowledge about practice development.

> I grew to appreciate the value of the practice development and the way it helped me to keep track of the journey, challenge different perspectives, develop new skills, facilitate reflection and bring about the changes needed. (McCormack et al., 2010)

And so you are clear, the activities themselves will help you develop your way of working or your practice. They get you, the people you care for and the care team into action together. We have also given you choices of activities so that you can find the ones that fit with what you do and your setting. But remember, working with this resource is likely to take you into new and sometimes difficult ground, so we provide ideas and suggest where you might get further local support.

In summary, using the resource can benefit you, the care team, people who receive care, families and others. It will also benefit the organisation's business because achieving more person-centred workplaces through practice development improves effectiveness. However, the resource needs to be introduced with care and sensitivity where staff or managers are not familiar with practice development or workplace learning.

How can this resource be used in your workplace?

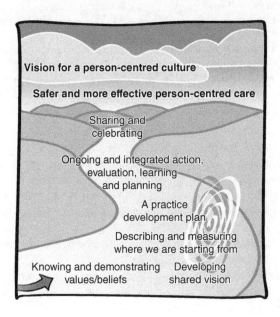

Vision for a person-centred culture

Safer and more effective person-centred care

Sharing and celebrating

Ongoing and integrated action, evaluation, learning and planning

A practice development plan

Describing and measuring where we are starting from

Knowing and demonstrating values/beliefs

Developing shared vision

Fig. 1.1 The key steps of the practice development journey.

The resources follow the steps of the practice development journey (see Figure 1.1). They are set out in the following chapters, each with a different theme.

Chapter 2	Knowing and demonstrating values and beliefs about person-centred care
Chapter 3	Developing a shared vision for person-centred care
Chapter 4	Introduction to measuring progress and evaluation
Chapter 5	Getting started together: Measuring and evaluating where we are now
Chapter 6	A practice development plan
Chapter 7	Mini-projects: Ongoing and integrated action, evaluation, learning and planning
Chapter 8	Learning in the workplace
Chapter 9	What if . . .? When things don't go so well
Chapter 10	Practice development as a continuous process (also see the companion website at **www.wiley.com/go/practicedevelopment/workbook**
Bonus online chapter	Sharing and celebrating (available at **www.wiley.com/go/practicedevelopment/workbook**)

Within each chapter there are materials (e.g. templates, posters, guidance, handouts, learning activities and tools) that you can use in your practice development work. Some of these are in the book itself as they are integral to the learning activity set out, whilst others are located on the companion website to this book. Visit **www.wiley.com/go/ practicedevelopment/workbook** where you can find these additional resources to help you with your work.

We imagine that those who will be leading, coordinating and facilitating the development of practice will be the people who familiarise themselves in more depth with what the resource offers. Then, use and direct others to sections and materials that will be useful to them at that time.

We stress here, again, that this resource is a vast treasure trove of materials. This is because practice development is a multi-faceted process and involves many different aspects. We have kept it big to provide you with a wide range and diversity of materials to choose from to find the best fit. We do not expect that you will use anywhere near all the materials. Neither do we expect you to read the resource as if it was a book. You can think of it as being a collection of assets and learning activities that you can draw on at certain times during your work over the coming years. It is more about cherry-picking what you need at different times. We suggest, therefore, do not look at it all at once. Then you and others will not be overloaded! To be able to cherry-pick, you will need to familiarise yourself with the resource. You can do this as follows.

- View the list of *Contents* that appears at the front of the book. This list will show you the structure and themes.
- Print out or look at the initial summary and introduction to each chapter. In each of these, there is a sub-section, 'Resources in this chapter'.
- Read these introductions and sub-sections – to give you a 'map' of the resource.
- Identify which guides, handouts, activities and tools look appealing: at the front of each guide there is a summary of what it is and who it is for.
- Use the list of *Contents* to find out which page they are on.
- Visit the companion website **www.wiley.com/go/practicedevelopment/workbook** to see the additional resources and print off those that are most useful to you for the activity/activities you are engaging in.

The ways you use the materials will vary according to what the resource is, your experience and skills, the kind of work you are doing, who you are helping or working with and so on. For example, some resources may help you to plan out a brief 15 minute learning activity or meeting in the overlap period between shifts, so that the structure, content and processes are more effective. In some cases, they can help you to take risks in trying out new ways of helping people to learn and change. They may even help you when you are feeling 'stuck' for what to do! Looking through these resources may help you to generate new ideas.

You may decide to find a learning buddy, someone in the team who you trust and who you think will help you to think about your work and give you honest feedback about your learning. Buddies are there for each other, so you could do the same for them or another colleague. For more ideas about learning with a buddy, see Chapter 8. Alternatively, if you have a clinical supervisor, this person can help you with your learning as part of your clinical supervision.

You might like to buy yourself a nice, small notebook (or decorate a more functional one!) to use for these and all the learning activities in this resource.

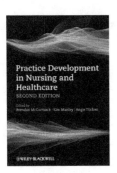

You are free to copy parts of the material for your own and your team's use, except where indicated otherwise. You can make multiple or partial photocopies of the materials for your own use/use with colleagues. Also, you can adapt them to your own situation unless it is stated that they cannot be changed in any way.

If you adapt any materials, please acknowledge the original source by adding, for example: 'adapted from Dewing, McCormack & Titchen (2013) *Practice Development Workbook for Nursing, Health and Social Care Teams*, John Wiley & Sons, Oxford.

If the materials already have a reference in their title, for example: Claims, concerns and issues: An evaluation tool for working with stakeholders (Guba & Lincoln, 1989), please leave in the reference (e.g. Guba & Lincoln (1989)) and add 'adapted from Dewing, McCormack & Titchen (2013) *Practice Development Workbook for Nursing, Health and Social Care Teams*, John Wiley & Sons, Oxford.'

To use materials from the print book outside of the workplace/care setting, please visit www.wiley.com and request permissions.

You will also find some further tools and resources (such as presentations) on this website: **www.wiley.com/go/ practicedevelopment/workbook**

That is the introduction to this collection of resources. Please feel free to browse through the rest of the resource. However, if you are interested in finding out more about practice development please continue reading as we set the scene by discussing a little more about practice development. This is a brief overview of the subject area that will give you some essential insights and understandings. This subject matter is elaborated on in *Practice Development in Nursing and Healthcare* (McCormack et al., 2013), which directly complements this resource. You might like to have it available to you and your team as an additional resource and a source of detailed information to answer questions and issues that arise as you progress with your practice development journey.

What is practice development?

> Practice development is a continuous journey of developing, and innovating in care settings, so that patients/residents, families and the team engage with each other in person-centred ways.
>
> This engagement is brought about by teams developing their knowledge and skills and changing the culture and organisation of care.
>
> It is helped to happen by the team working with systematic and continuous processes of development and evaluation that involve and include the views, experiences and needs of patients/residents, families, the team and others.
>
> Adapted from Garbett & McCormack (2002)

Practice development begins with a shared vision and purpose about the development journey to be taken. Visions of this kind are based on people's values. Values are buried very deep in us and in the workplace culture of our care settings and care homes. They are often invisible, so if we want to be effective as a team in bringing about change together, we need to bring everyone's values out into the open. To begin practice development we must:

- make our own values clear to ourselves and others because it is our values that drive the kind of care we give or would like to give (if all the things like lack of time and money that stop us from doing so were removed).
- be respectful of values that are different from our own. When we can talk together about what we value and what we want to create together, this talk gives us the opportunity to find some common ground about what the vision for the development or the direction of travel could be.
- agree the common ground and shared interests. This common ground or shared values is the very foundation for the practice development journey as you can see in Figure 1.1. These shared values will inform the development of the vision of the care home that you will be creating in Chapters 2 and 3 of this resource.

And again, if you can imagine Figure 1.2 as three round blocks stacked one on top of the other and you are looking from the top, then it is the shared values and vision that are the firm foundation. The main effort in practice development comes when we start to seriously examine how the values we talk about are or are not put into action every day.

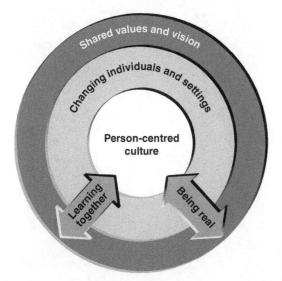

Fig. 1.2 Practice development (adapted from Garbett & McCormack, 2002).

It gets more complex though, because not everyone in the care setting or home will have the same values or the same priorities – because we are all different people. For example, if you value offering patients/residents care that meets their needs, as they see them, and time and again you observe that people are not getting that kind of care, then there is a gap. When there is a gap between the talked about values and the values really being put into action, it is unlikely a shared vision of a person-centred culture will become real in any significant way (see the top of the stack or centre of Figure 1.2). It is also unlikely to become real, if you or other team members prize or value efficiency and getting through the work (tasks) quickly above being with people and being person-centred.

Working and learning together in a practice development way, these differences are acknowledged and we try to find the values that we do share. We identify where we are prepared to give ground and move towards each others' values. The important principle to establish is that everyone is prepared to look at or relook at their values and how they live them in the way they work. Making a vision come 'alive' nearly always means that we have to be willing to change ourselves and our workplace settings in some way (see the second ring in Figure 1.2). We do that by learning together and being real, that is, by being ourselves rather than by hiding behind a role or wearing a mask (shown by the arrows moving from shared vision to a person-centred culture in Figure 1.2). How this is actually done is the content of the rest of this resource.

The principles of practice development work

When we begin building on Figure 1.2, we see the principles of practice development as:

- based on working towards a shared common vision.
- a continuous process of improvement and innovation towards:
  - increased effectiveness in person-centred care
  - a longer-term sustainable transformation of the culture and organisation of care.
- brought about by teams developing their knowledge and skills through reflection and work-based learning.
- helped by teams being committed to systematic, rigorous and continuous processes of change. These processes of change aim to free us from the obstacles inside us and outside us in the care setting (these obstacles get in the way of us achieving our shared vision).
- being real. We've made this adaption to the original model and included this because we feel that being real is essential to developing person-centredness. We need to learn to be authentic and genuine in how we relate to others in order for more meaningful relationships to thrive.
- reflecting the perspectives of patients/residents and families.

This last principle means that we need to be learning with and from patients/residents and families. This leads us to the person-centred framework that also underpins this resource.

The person-centred practice framework

> ### So what is person-centred working ?
>
> We suggest that it is a way of working that helps patients/residents to maintain or enhance their identity and freedom, feel included and attached and be provided with comfort and occupation. This involves being treated respectfully as a person, participating in decision-making about care, being part of and contributing to the care setting and being involved in shared decision-making.
>
> It is 'an approach to work or practice established through the formation and fostering of therapeutic relationships between all care providers, older people and others significant to them in their lives. It is underpinned by values of respect for persons, individual right to self-determination, mutual respect and understanding. It is enabled by cultures of empowerment that foster continuous approaches to practice development.' (McCormack et al., 2010: 25)

However, to create the conditions for such work for all patients/residents, we need to understand this complexity in preparation for the whole practice development journey. This journey might include, of course, the development of your skills for working with families and patients/residents who are living with a variety of conditions.

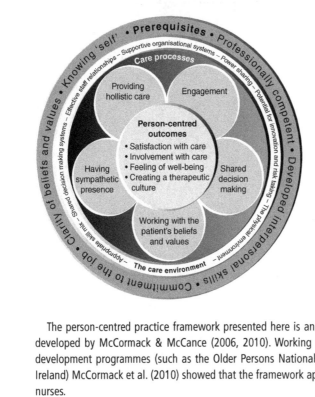

Fig. 1.3 The person-centred practice framework (McCormack & McCance, 2010).

The person-centred practice framework presented here is an adaptation of the Person-centred Nursing Framework developed by McCormack & McCance (2006, 2010). Working with the original framework in a number of practice development programmes (such as the Older Persons National Practice Development Programme in the Republic of Ireland) McCormack et al. (2010) showed that the framework applied to all health and social care workers and not just nurses.

> The Framework has four parts:
> * prerequisites, which are the qualities and skills of the care worker/team member;
> * the care environment, which focuses on the setting in which care is delivered;
> * person-centred processes, which focus on delivering care through a range of activities;
> * expected outcomes, which are the results of effective person-centred practice.

The relationship between the parts of the framework is shown in Figure 1.3, that is, to reach the centre of the framework, the prerequisites must first be considered and then the care environment, both of which are necessary in providing effective care through the care processes. This ordering, leads to more person-centred care processes and ultimately to the achievement of the outcomes – the central component of the framework. This is not to suggest that you can't think or bring about changes to the care setting before doing work on the qualities and skills of the care worker, because in reality these activities often happen at the same time. However, basically it is a way of thinking about all the necessary parts for creating a person-centred culture, that is, we need to:

- work on having the best team in place;
- strive to make the environment of care work to support person-centred principles;
- engage with patients/residents in particular ways.

All these things together create a person-centred culture and help us achieve person-centred outcomes for patients/residents, care staff, teams and organisations.

The prerequisites focus on the characteristics and qualities of the care worker. They include:

- being competent to do the job having developed interpersonal skills;
- being committed to the job;
- being clear about beliefs and values;
- knowing who you are as a person (what you believe in, knowing what you feel strongly about etc).

The care environment focuses on the setting in which care is delivered and includes:

- having the right staff skill mix and staffing levels to be able to deliver person-centred care;
- facilitation of discussions between those involved in the care of patients/residents (including family members) to:
  - develop effective staff relationships
  - to share power as a team and with patients/residents and families;
- organisational systems that are supportive
- potential for innovation and risk taking.

Supportive organisational systems acknowledge the incredible influence that organisational culture can have on (1) the quality of care delivered and (2) the freedom afforded to care staff to work autonomously, be innovative and take assessed risks. Finally, we know that the physical environment can have an impact on being able to work in a person-centred way – for example, it is easier to plan individualised washing and dressing when a service or facility has en-suite rooms, rather than bathrooms shared between a group of patients/residents.

Person-centred processes specifically focus on the patient/resident, describing core aspects of person-centred practice in the context of care delivery through a range of activities that make person-centred practice real. Working with patients/residents' beliefs and values reinforces one of the fundamental principles of person-centred care, which places importance on developing a clear picture of what the patient/resident values about his/her life and how he/she makes sense of what is happening.

Working with patients/residents' beliefs and values is closely linked to shared decision-making. This focuses on team members helping patients/residents participate by providing information and integrating it into the way things are usually done. However, this is dependent on systems that facilitate shared decision-making (the care environment). This must involve a process of negotiation. This negotiation must take account of the patient/resident's values to form a sound basis for decision-making. The success of this negotiation rests on successful communication. Having sympathetic presence as a care worker means showing that you recognise the patient/resident's uniqueness and value in the way you are with them and the way you work with them. Finally, providing holistic care by competent care workers is essential because it is a 'way in' to carrying out person-centred processes and to achieving person-centred outcomes.

Outcomes are the results expected from effective person-centred practice and include:

- satisfaction with care;
- involvement in care;
- feeling of well-being;
- creating a therapeutic environment.

Patient and resident satisfaction reflects the ways in which a patient/resident evaluates their care experiences. Involvement in care is the outcome expected as a result of participating in shared decision-making processes. A feeling of well-being indicates that the patient/resident feels valued and includes mental and physical well-being.

Finally, a therapeutic environment is one where decision-making is shared, staff relationships are collaborative, leadership is effective and innovative practices are supported – this is the ultimate outcome for teams working to develop a workplace that is person-centred.

To learn more about practice development and person-centred practice, read relevant chapters in *Practice Development in Nursing and Healthcare* (McCormack et al., 2013). This book contains up-to-date thinking on practice development and person-centred practice that is illustrated with real-life examples.

You will have noticed that in both these frameworks, clarity of values and beliefs is at the foundation (the outer ring). For this reason, Chapter 2 focuses on knowing and demonstrating our values about person-centred care. Chapter 3 will help you to start to build a vision for person-centred practice based on the values that you and the people who live, work and visit the care home hold.

So now it's over to you to make use of the resource!

Useful websites and resources (also see Chapters 3, 5, 8, 10 & bonus online chapter and for Frequently Asked Questions, see Chapter 9)

 For ease of use, this section is also available on the companion website: **www.wiley.com/go/practicedevelopment/workbook**

1. **Department of Health** offers a range of resources on its website relevant to all settings and health-care groups such as people living with dementia (www.dh.gov.uk, http://dementia.dh.gov.uk).
   There is also an Information Portal with resources for implementing the National Dementia Strategy.

   Quality outcomes for people with dementia: building on the work of the National Dementia Strategy (www.dh.gov.uk/en/Publicationsandstatistics/Publications/PublicationsPolicyAndGuidance/DH_119827)

   Who cares? Information & support for the carers of people with dementia (www.dh.gov.uk/prod_consum_dh/groups/dh_digitalassets/@dh/@en/documents/digitalasset/dh_078091.pdf)

2. **NHS National Institute for Health & Clinical Excellence (NICE)**
   NICE quality standards set out aspirational, but achievable, descriptions of high-quality and cost-effective patient care. The standards cover the treatment and prevention of different diseases and common conditions. Drawing on the best available evidence, such as NICE guidance and other sources of evidence that have been accredited by NHS Evidence (www.evidence.nhs.uk/default.aspx), the standards are developed in collaboration with NHS and social care professionals and service users, and address three dimensions of quality:
   • clinical effectiveness;
   • patient safety;
   • patient experience.
   There is also, for example, a dementia quality standard. (www.nice.org.uk/aboutnice/qualitystandards)

3. **NHS Improving Quality**
   NHS Improving Quality works to improve health outcomes across England by providing improvement and change expertise –
   See more at: www.nhsiq.nhs.uk/#sthash.iNh0jDgo.dpuf
   This site offers short videos of patients' stories of their experiences of health care in many different fields of clinical practice. In this chapter we show you how you can use these videos in your workplace to start you off on your practice development journey.

4. **The King's Fund**

    The King's Fund aims to understand how the health-care system in England can be improved. The organisation works with individuals and organisations to shape policy, transform services and bring about changes that will result in changes of behaviour.

    This website contains reports and strategy documents that may be useful for NHS service and care home managers who are leading strategic developments. It includes information about the educational programmes offered to senior managers and those aspiring to become such managers (www.kingsfund.org.uk/).

5. **England Centre for Practice Development**

    The Centre has a commitment to increase scholarly activities and research in practice development to improve patient and service user experiences of care. It is hosted and based at Canterbury Christ Church University, and its members are part of the International Practice Development Collaborative (IPDC). Whether you are leading a practice development project, want to increase your skills in practice development, or are interested in partnership working within practice and service development, the ECPD can support you for the benefit of your practice and the practice of others (www.canterbury.ac.uk/health/EnglandCentreforPracticeDevelopment/Home.aspx).

6. **Person-centred Practice Research Centre (PcPRC), Institute of Nursing and Health Research**

    The vision for the PcPRC is to be a world-leading centre in research and development that has as its focus the enhancement of knowledge and expertise in person-centred practice by:

    - providing safe, supportive and challenging thinking spaces;
    - working openly;
    - keeping practice at the core of their work;
    - valuing individual strengths, experiences and commitments;
    - nurturing newness and individual development;
    - celebrating achievements.

    There is a list of publications with abstracts and resources/tools you can download from the website (www.science.ulster.ac.uk/inr/pcp.php).

7. **Foundation of Nursing Studies – Centre for Nursing Innovation**

    In the Centre for Nursing Innovation you will find:

    - a library of information about leading and facilitating innovation and change;
    - A free access e-journal: The International Practice Development Journal (see 11 further on);
    - a learning zone containing useful tools and resources;
    - a common room where you can interact with others;
    - programmes of support, facilitation and funding.

    (www.fons.org)

8. **The Patients Association**

    The Patients Association listens to patients and speaks up for change. The organisation is perhaps best known for capturing stories about health care from over thousands of patients, family members and carers every year. They use this knowledge to campaign for real improvements to health and social care services across the UK. The association has also produced a number of research reports including our two reports on poor care in hospital: 'Listen to Patients, Speak up for Change', 'Patients not Numbers, People not Statistics', our report on the Health and Social Care Bill 'PAUSE: Patients Association Urges Serious Examination', and various others including 'Public Attitudes to Pain', 'Meaningful and comparable information? Tissue Viability Nursing Services and Pressure Ulcers' and 'Malnutrition in the Hospital and Community Setting'.

    You will find booklets, publications and more information on this website (www.patients-association.com).

9. **Picker Institute**

    The Picker Institute is an independent non-profit organisation dedicated to the principles of patient-centred care. In cooperation with a range of educational institutions and other organisations and individuals, the Picker Institute sponsors awards, research and education to promote patient-centred care and the patient-centred care movement.

    Eight principles for patient-centred care are offered on this website, which you may find useful for discussion in your workplace (www.pickerinstitute.org).

10. **Kissing it Better**

    Kissing it Better is about the little things that make the world of difference to health care. The organisation focuses on improving practical concerns such as good communication, appetising food, comfort and surroundings – things that show both patients and their carers that the traditional values of health-care providers are central to good care. *Kissing it Better* offers an easy-to-use, on-line 'suggestion box' of what has been shown by experience to work. The website offers good ideas for transforming patient care. Simple but powerful ways of being person-centred in the everyday things of patient/resident care in all fields of practice could be used to inspire changes in your setting/home (www.kissingitbetter.co.uk).

11. **International Practice Development Journal (IPDJ)**

    The International Practice Development Journal is a free online journal with a vision, over the next five years, of becoming the first choice publication for academics and practitioners working in the practice development field internationally. The aim is to publish material that challenges assumptions and provokes new visions and ideas, helping health-care workers engage in dialogue about the contribution practice development makes to health-care services and academia. There are an increasing number of reflective articles by practitioners on their experience of doing practice development.

    Just visit the website of the Foundation of Nursing Studies (www.fons.org) and sign up for free access. Also see the other pages on the Foundation of Nursing Studies website for ideas and possible sources of project funding for practice development work.

12. **Opening doors on creativity: Resources to awaken creative working**

    This resource offered by the Royal College of Nursing (RCN), is for health-care practitioners who have a responsibility for, or an interest in, systematic practice development and its associated areas, such as evidence-based practice, clinical leadership or clinical governance. The resource could provide a 'spark' to ignite your enthusiasm for using more creative ways of thinking about practice development, develop your practical skills and confidence with creativity, and enable you to facilitate learning activities for others using new skills and creative facilitation. *Opening doors* combines creative activities, imagery, practical ideas and mini-case examples. It seeks to extend further the ability of practitioners to liberate their own feelings and thinking and use innovative strategies with others, for the purposes of practice transformation within person-centred, evidence-based care. The resource in PDF form can be accessed by Googling the title or going through the RCN website (www.rcn.org.uk).

13. **Health Service Executive (HSE), Ireland**

    In 2010, the HSE published a guide developed from the Irish programme, entitled 'Enhancing Care for Older People – A Guide to Practice Development Processes to Support and Enhance Care in Residential Settings for Older People'. We recommend Sections 4 and 5 of the Ireland guide as complementary to this section here.

    You can access the complete programme report and a workplace learning resource from the Lenus website (www.lenus.ie).

14. **Age UK** also offers a range of publications, information, guides and factsheets for older people in general. In particular, this document might be useful for you to get at the perspective of people who live in care homes and their families as you work with this resource. (www.ageuk.org.uk).

15. **Social Care Institute for Excellence (SCIE)**

    This is an excellent website that is well worthwhile browsing for inspiration. For example, it has a number of videos about care of people and being person-centred (they call it 'personalisation'). These videos can be used as learning resources (www.scie.org.uk/socialcaretv/topic.asp?guid=6ddc31cf-a355-46cf-9fce -2685b51272d3).

16. **Places to Flourish**

    This beautiful resource has been developed to support continued quality improvement in residential care services for older people. The resource builds on the principles of the Teaghlach model and the National Person Centred Care Programme and other national quality initiatives in Ireland. Its intention is to encourage innovation and an improved experience of living and working in all public and private residential care settings (www.placestoflourish.org).

17. **Relatives & Residents Association**

    The Relatives & Residents Association offers help to residents in care homes and their families in three key areas: a helpline, campaigning and resources and projects. You can download posters, leaflets and newsletters for free from this website (www.relres.org).

18. *My* **Home Life** – a new initiative aimed at improving the quality of life of those who are living, dying, visiting and working in care homes for older people (www.myhomelifemovement.org.uk).

    My **Home Life** aims to celebrate existing best practice in care homes and promote care homes as a positive option for some older people. The *My* **Home Life** team offers a range of resources, events, initiatives and other activities. Their research has identified eight practice themes, which together form a vision for care homes. There are videos illustrating these themes that you can download and use as learning resources.

Chapter 2   Knowing and Demonstrating Values and Beliefs about Person-Centred Care

Contents

Introduction

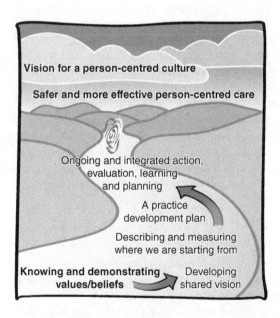

Fig. 2.1 A step on the practice development journey: Knowing and demonstrating values and beliefs.

Chapter 2 explains how to get started on developing practice in your care setting/care home. To begin requires that everyone becomes more aware of the values and beliefs they hold about providing care and service for patients/residents. We explain that this will lead eventually to creating a shared vision in the setting. In this chapter, we show you how you can become more aware of your values and beliefs and how you can share them with others – the talking. In the next chapter, we show you how you can create a shared vision in your setting – the doing.

Practice Development Workbook for Nursing, Health and Social Care Teams, First Edition. Jan Dewing, Brendan McCormack, and Angie Titchen.
© 2014 John Wiley & Sons, Ltd. Published 2014 by John Wiley & Sons, Ltd.
Companion website: www.wiley.com/go/practicedevelopment/workbook

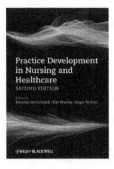

The materials in this chapter are suitable for staff across all care settings to choose from except for the guidance sheets on how to run some of the activities. We suggest who these sheets might be useful for for people acting as facilitators of activities with others. We indicate which materials are also useful for patients/residents, families, friends and volunteers.

You might like to read Chapter 1 of *Practice Development in Nursing and Healthcare* (McCormack et al., 2013) in which Brendan McCormack, Kim Manley and Angie Titchen put practice development and person-centred practice in context. This might help you understand the bigger picture pertaining to the need for practice development and how person-centredness and practice development are connected with each other.

Making our values and beliefs clear is essential, because they underpin all we do in our practice. This is why clarity of beliefs and values is a prerequisite for person-centred practice (see Figure 1.3 in Chapter 1). So clarifying values and beliefs and agreeing those that you share with others in your care setting or care home is the first step in collaborative practice development work. In Chapter 1, we said that practice development is based on working towards a shared common vision.

You can create a shared or common vision from the shared values and beliefs of patients/residents, families and others (including carers, catering and cleaning workers, managers, leaders and volunteers). Thus, in practice development, activities to make values and beliefs clear often blend into activities for developing a shared vision. However, in this resource we have separated them out into this chapter and Chapter 3 so you can see clearly the activities to find out what the shared values and beliefs are and then what needs to be done to agree a shared vision.

Many organisations believe in having a clearly written philosophy or mission statement that sets out:

- aim(s) of the organisation;
- the organisation's primary stakeholders: patients/clients/customers, shareholders, congregation etc.;
- How the organisation provides value to these stakeholders, for example by offering specific types of products and/ or services.

The critical factor is that a mission or vision statement should influence every aspect of the service or care home and make it possible to measure how well the service or home is living up to its standards at any time.

Plough the furrow and plant the seed at the same time   Thus, having a mission or vision statement is more than words on paper – the statement needs to be really owned, lived and experienced by those who live and work there. As you work through the activities in this chapter (and the rest of the resource), you will be learning how to include people so they *really* feel this ownership. Including people in practice development and helping them to collaborate and participate in it, requires person-centred skills. These are the same fundamental skills that are needed for person-centred care of individual patients/residents, carers and families. So the activities in this entire resource help you with two things at the same time.

Resources in this chapter

Learning activities – these activities will prepare you and others for the values clarification activity below. They will begin to bring to everyone's attention the values that are operating now in the setting and those we might like to see in the future. **There are a range of activities for you to choose from.** You do NOT need to do all of them. They progress from ones that you can do alone or with a colleague to informal small groups, which don't need a skilled facilitator, and formal group activities, which do. You may decide to ask your learning buddy or clinical supervisor to support you, help you to think about your work and give you honest feedback about your learning. For more ideas about learning with a buddy, see Chapter 8. Remember that a notebook might be useful for these and all the learning activities in this resource.

- **Individual values and beliefs** – these have been designed to get you thinking about what you really value, what really matters to you in the care/service you offer. They are done by yourself or with one other person.
- **Group/team values and beliefs** – together with others, activities are offered to help a group to identify the values and beliefs that influence their care/service as a group.
- **Organisational values and beliefs** – together with others, this activity helps groups to identify the values and beliefs that underpin the whole care setting/home or organisation.

- **Scenarios for discussion groups** – about 'lip service' or the gaps between what we say are our values and those that we and others actually experience being put into action.
- **How to feature values and beliefs in the care setting** – this resource offers other suggestions about raising awareness about values and beliefs and the need for values clarification across the care setting/care home as a preparation to creating a shared vision and common purpose for practice development in the setting or home. A quick evaluation tool to raise awareness is offered on the companion website (**www.wiley.com/go/practicedevelopment/workbook**) to further raise awareness.

Values and beliefs template – this template consists of five statements that people in your care setting respond to. See below for more detail about how the activity can be facilitated.

This activity to clarify values and beliefs can be carried out on whatever topic you need. This can be any aspect of work (or life!) in the care setting, and the ways you work. The template leaves a blank for you to fill in whatever topic you are exploring, such as:

- the patients/residents' day;
- providing care in people's own homes;
- admission to care (moving into a care home);
- pre- and post-operative recovery;
- social activities;
- leadership;
- helping people;
- learning at work;
- person-centred care;
- your role;
- privacy/dignity;
- pain management;
- working with families.

Decide what it is that is most urgent or central to your work and purpose. It's important not to be too ambitious by undertaking a values clarification activity in more than one area at a time, as this will lead to confusion rather than clarity.

Values and beliefs clarification method – next we show you a method you and your team can use to explore values and beliefs. There are also alternative and complementary ways that you can deliver this activity according to how much time you have, for example, using pictures to help think about the ideas on the template first, or using painting to create a visual image. If you or anyone you work with has any creative tendencies or abilities then they may help you come up with some other ideas.

Most if not all the activities in this chapter can be offered to students and other learners on placement.

In the next section, some creative methods are included to give you an idea of the possibilities. The guidance here, however, focuses on undertaking the activity in the simplest and shortest time within your day-to-day work.

In Chapter 9, there are Frequently Asked Questions that you might find helpful *when the possibility of developing practice in your setting is first discussed.*

Reflection on my own values and beliefs about the care/service I give or receive

Learning activity for patients/residents, families, friends, care staff, newly employed team members, volunteers and students/learners

The activity only requires a simple pack/collection of picture cards, such as a set of postcards or greeting cards that you collect for yourself or that you buy in somewhere like the *personal development* section of a book shop or on the Internet. Alternatively, you could get together a collection of photos you have taken or cut pictures out of magazines.

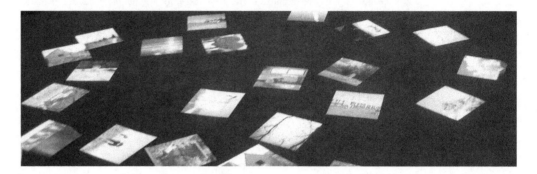

The purpose of the activity is to help you begin to express, for yourself, the things that you value and are really important to you in terms of the care setting/care home. This activity can help remind you what matters to you and how you can feel about working, receiving care or living in a care setting/care home.

You will need:

- 15 minutes;
- a copy of this sheet of instructions;
- a quiet room or space in the care setting/care home (remember to consider using outside spaces such as a garden if there is one) where you won't be disturbed or questioned about what you are doing;
- a notebook or piece of paper and pen;
- a pack of cards.

Key activities

Lay out the cards on the floor, ground or table, face up. Then sit quietly for a moment, giving yourself time to make a clear break from what you have just been doing. Take a few deep breaths and relax as you breathe out. Then choose the pictures (as many as you want) that attract you. You don't have to have any reason at all, at this point, other than you notice them more than the others. (3 mins)

Now lay out the cards/pictures you have chosen, and really look at them. Ask yourself: (5 mins)

- What do I like about this card/picture and why?
- Does anything about the card/picture symbolise or represent something that I value?
- What does the card/picture say about people?
- Does the card/picture tell me anything about what I value about the care/service that I give or I receive in this care setting/care home?
- What is it that matters in the care/service I give or receive?

If you work across several care settings such as in many community services then choose one setting that you would like to focus on.

Write down in your notebook or on a piece of paper the things that really matter to you; the things that you really value. To help you remember for future activities on other days, you might like to take a photo, quickly sketch the card(s) that helped you to discover these things in your notebook, or keep the cards/pictures beside your notes, if they belong to you.

Think about what this activity has shown you in relation to your values and beliefs about person-centred care. You might like to summarise your values and beliefs on the worksheet later in this section.

An alternative way of doing this activity   A different way of expressing or naming your values and beliefs for yourself can be done in the same way and time as above, but instead of using a pack of cards, you can use:

- the contents of your pockets or bag or
- an object from home or work that you think captures or symbolises something that matters to you (the real you).

When you ask yourself the above questions, just replace the words 'card/picture' for whatever you are using.

You can also do these activities with a learning buddy/supervisor   You choose your cards or object and reflect alone on the questions and then share with each other what the cards or object mean to you. The idea is that talking about them often increases our understanding further. The buddy/supervisor listens and only asks questions to clarify things for you. There is no discussion, at this early stage, as the purpose for now is to help each other to talk about things that are often invisible in our practice or so taken for granted that they are rarely spoken. If you discover differences in your values, just recognise it. The worksheet will help you record what you are learning about yourself.
Think about:

- What you shared in common and what differences you had?
- How can you work together on the things you had in common?
- How can you better understand each other's differences?

If you have 20–25 minutes of time available, then you could try the next activity.

Going for a reflective walk on your own or with someone else

> Learning activity for care team members (including newly employed team members and students/learners on placement), patients/residents, families, friends and volunteers

The purpose of this activity is to help you identify, for yourself or for example with the help of your buddy/supervisor, the things that you value and are really important to you in terms of your own work in the care setting or care home. The idea is that you take a quiet walk on your own or together (not stopping to talk to anyone on the way). Given the busy environment of many care settings, you might consider walking around the grounds or the immediate surroundings where you work, whatever they might be. Or if you are a community worker you might decide to do this alone, on the way to or from work if it involves walking at some point.
You will need:

- 20 minutes (if walking alone) or 30 minutes (if you walk with someone else);
- a copy of this sheet of instructions;
- a pen and a small notebook or piece of paper folded into four (tucked into your pocket if possible).

Key activities

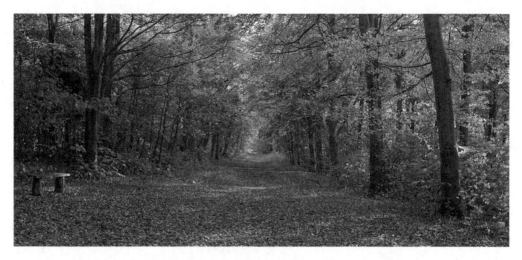

Source: © Jane Stokes (www.janestokes.com) 2014 All Rights Reserved.

When you have decided where you will go, pause for a moment or two before you set off to take a few deep breaths and let go of whatever thoughts are in your mind. You can do this 'letting go' by really looking around you, as if you had never seen these surroundings and things before. As you walk, notice what you really notice, what captures your attention, what you feel, and write these things down (a word, phrase or image) or sketch them roughly. There doesn't have to be any reason at all for what you notice. The important thing is that these particular things just happen to attract you. And it is this noticing that often reveals what we value even when we didn't know it ourselves! (10 mins)

After 10 or 15 minutes, sit down if you can and reflect on your own (or with your walking partner or buddy) on the words and images that might come to your mind by asking yourself (or each other) the following questions.

- What is it about these things that I/you have noticed that I/you value?
- How do I/you feel?
- What comes to my/your imagination about these things?
- Do these things symbolise or represent something that I/you value?
- Do they say anything about:
  - what I/you value about the care/service that I/you give in the care setting/care home
  - **or** what I/you value about the care/service that I/you receive?
- What is it that really matters in the care/service I/you give **or** receive? (takes approximately 5–10 mins)

This activity can be adapted for people with impaired senses, cognition and/or mobility.

Record any insights about your values that come up for you from this reflection in your notebook or on your paper and think about what they might mean for care and, especially, for care of people with dementia if there are any. Later, you might like to record them on your worksheet.

If you get the opportunity to carry out values and beliefs clarification work as a group (see later in this chapter), this activity may help you prepare for it.

Values and beliefs of the care setting

Learning activity for care staff, newly employed team members, students/ learners on placement and volunteers

The purpose of this learning activity is to experience the lived values and beliefs of your care setting from the perspective of a patient, resident or service user. You can do this by imagining that you are a patient, resident or user.

For example:

In the in-patient, out-patient or community service setting, you might be a person who is coming for the first time and is acutely aware of the setting.

In the care home, you might be a person in the initial stages of dementia coming along with someone, such as your daughter, son or friend to check out whether the care home might be suitable for you at some point in the future.

You will need:

- 20 minutes;
- to tell your colleagues what you (and your buddy if you are doing it together) are doing in advance and that the purpose is not to criticise them but to imagine what the setting might be like for patients/residents and their families;
- a copy of this sheet of instructions;
- notebook or paper and pen;
- camera (if you have one);
- the ward or service information materials or the care home promotional materials, for example, flyers, leaflets, information sheets.

Note: when using a camera you must not take photos of other people. Any photos you take must be used only for your learning needs and not shared with any other people. Please check your/the organisation's local policy.

Key activities

Look carefully around you as you come in the front entrance. What is your first impression? How do you feel as you enter? What can you hear? Is it welcoming? What do you see? Is there any signage? What is on the walls? How does it smell?

Walk around the setting or home, really looking at it from the point of view of being a patient or resident yourself or the relative/friend of a person you are visiting. Look at the fabric and furnishings of the building and at what patients/ residents are doing and how they are interacting. Feel the atmosphere.

Take pictures as you go.

Ask yourselves the following questions and make notes as you walk around:

- What do I really like about the setting?
- What do I really dislike about it?
- Would I really like to be cared for/live here?
- Would my care needs be met here?
- Would my day-to-day life needs be met here?
- What would staying or living here say about me?

Now find a quiet spot and look at promotional and information materials together.

- Do your observations, impressions and feelings match up to what the materials say about the setting or home and the care it provides patients/residents and families?

- Think about the values you see in these materials and those you saw actually demonstrated in the setting or home on that brief 'visit' to it in your learning activity.
- Make notes in response to these reflections or thoughts.
- If you have time at a later point, look up the Trust or organisation on the Internet – what can you find out about it?

Sharing your findings and learning from this activity can take place in a number of ways, for example:

- discussion with your buddy or another team member;
- in clinical supervision;
- in a team, staff or residents meeting;
- making a poster or collage (see Figure 2.2).

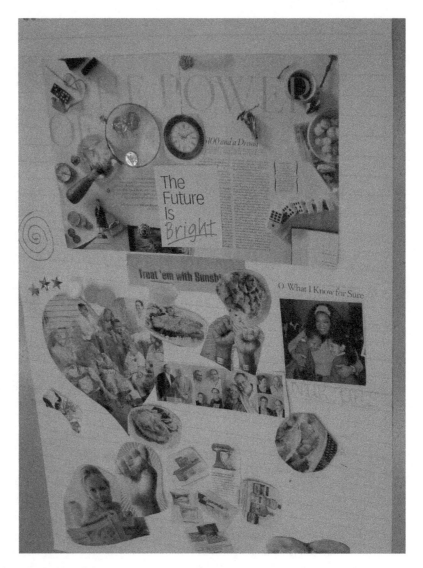

Fig. 2.2 Making a poster or collage.

There is now an observation method set up for adult and children's services in the NHS (in acute, mental health and community contexts) that aims to help teams find out more about patients' and families' first impressions of health-care settings. It is similar to the method we have just described. You could use similar principles to suit a care home. (www.institute.nhs.uk/.../15stepschallenge/15stepschallenge.html)

I can tell what kind of care my daughter is going to get within 15 steps of walking on to a ward.

(Quote from parent that sparked the 15 Steps Challenge)

Leaders' values and beliefs

> Learning activity for service/care home managers/team leaders, Matrons, heads of therapy departments, governance managers, trustees, executive members)

As a leader, you will be aware that you are central in setting the ethos and climate in the care setting/care home and that you are in an ideal position to demonstrate your values and beliefs about person-centred care. So, you may have already undertaken some of the above activities alone or with a buddy or contributed to group discussions, in order to become *more aware of* your own values and beliefs. However, simply knowing them is not enough.

The purpose of this learning activity is to help you become more intentional in *demonstrating* your beliefs and values in your work, so that you 'model the way' and the importance of doing so to teams. In day-to-day work, we can share the values shaping our observations and evaluations of what is going on.

For example, you have observed that a patient is being prevented from doing something. You raise this as a concern with staff, without blaming, and ask why it is so important to stop the person from doing what they were intending to do.

You follow this observation and short conversation by asking the team leader to facilitate a discussion with the care team on how similar situations might be better responded to differently and more in keeping with the team's stated values and beliefs.

We can also demonstrate our values if we speak about the values that influence our decision-making. For instance, let's take the case of a discussion between a care worker and a housekeeper about what to do about a difficulty that a patient/resident is having about the behaviour of a fellow patient/resident with dementia.

> That Mr Woods is just getting too much for everyone. He is stopping them enjoying their meals. He should be stopped from eating when they do.

In the course of the discussion, you might say that the values that need to guide a decision on what to do need to be person-centred – in relation to the person seen as causing 'the bother', as well as the other people involved. We must work on the basis that the person is experiencing distress and their needs must also be responded to in positive and caring ways (Department of Health, (2013).

You suggest that a middle way must be found together with the patients/residents concerned and listen to what team members have to say.

In discussing the values of all those involved, you and the housekeeper identify a plan of action that helps the person with dementia to continue to have their meals without undue disruption by or to others. So you are demonstrating, in addition to your valuing of person-centredness, the value of shared decision-making by patients/residents and staff.

For the activity, you will need:

- internet access;
- a quiet space to sit and reflect;
- a notebook or paper and pen.

Key activities

Choose a situation that you were part of in your workplace and that you feel went really well. Reflect on the key values and beliefs that you demonstrated in this situation. Make notes as you reflect.

When you are ready, ask yourself the following questions, as a leader, and make notes.

- What impact are my values and beliefs having on team members, patients/residents and families?
- Do I talk to team members in a way that demonstrates what I value and believe in (whatever it is)?
- What opportunities do I take in the working day to demonstrate my values?
- Are there any other opportunities I could take, like shift handovers, meetings or tea breaks to make my values and beliefs clearer to team members?
- What are the values expressed in the workplace (for example, furnishings, decor and accessories), promotional materials, welcome packs, information sheets and posters that we have on display?

- Are we true to these values in the service(s) we provide?

Record any insights that emerge for you and think about what you might do with them, for example:

- presenting an issue for group discussion;
- creating opportunities to share your values and beliefs with team members;
- encouraging staff to express their values in shift handovers/work planning;
- being more visible to have conversations with others;
- helping to raise the profile of values and beliefs in the workplace (see next resource);
- rethinking promotional material and posters on display and so on.

Look at the handout on 'How to feature values and beliefs in your work around the care setting/care home' later in this chapter as you consider any action planning.

Sheet 2.1: Worksheet for recording learning activities with a buddy: Values and beliefs about . . . . care

The purpose of this worksheet is to help you record the work you do with your buddy or a fellow worker as you:

- get to know your own values and beliefs about . . . .;
- better understand how you are showing these values and beliefs in your work with people who are living with the condition you specify;
- become more aware if and when you are not living up to your values and beliefs about . . . . care.

Date: _____   Buddy/Supervisor: _____   Activity: _____

The three most important values and beliefs I have are:

_____
_____
_____

The key thing that I have learned today about demonstrating my values and beliefs is:

_____
_____
_____

In relation to living up to my values and beliefs, what I have learned is:

_____
_____
_____

The thing that stands out for me about others' values and beliefs is:

_____
_____
_____

Action: My actions to take before I meet with my buddy/supervisor again are:

_____
_____
_____

The most important thing that I have learned about person-centred care today is:

_____
_____
_____

Summary

My values and beliefs about person-centred care are: (you can add to this list after each activity as you become more aware of what they are and how you show them in your work)

_____
_____
_____
_____
_____
_____
_____
_____
_____
_____

Sheet 2.2: Discussion groups

Learning activity suitable for everyone in the care team

Discussions with some kind of trigger can result in very lively and useful learning by groups and teams. Discussions can be carried out, informally, in 20 minute time slots – for example, in a shift overlap period or during visiting. The role of leading the discussion can be rotated with the lead choosing the scenario or trigger to get the conversation going. A variety of scenarios and triggers are suggested on the companion website (**www.wiley.com/go/ practicedevelopment/workbook**). Here we offer guidance on how to get the best out of the discussion. In addition, we suggest how you can source your own triggers or materials for learning, for your own particular profession, field of practice and country. Of course, the discussion leader may decide to use a trigger based on an issue or something that has happened in the home. In this case, the session is not a blaming session. It is a conversation to try and understand what has happened and to agree a plan for what happens next. Further help on asking questions and helping people to reflect on their practice is offered in Chapter 8.

You will need:

- a space or room big enough depending on how many of you can get together at one time and the amount of space required (e.g. for wheelchairs);
- a small group of between 3 and 8 people, which may be a mix of team members, patients/residents, families and volunteers;
- a circle of chairs;
- a trigger or scenario – you may need to prepare or download the trigger in advance and copy it for people to read in advance;
- a computer if you are going to show a small video;
- prepare a focus for the discussion and some questions to get the discussion going;
- a scribe – best to ask someone in advance of the discussion to write up the key points on a flipchart;
- a flipchart or large piece of paper stuck on the wall, and pens to write up the key points and agreed actions.

Key activities A discussion has a beginning, middle and end.

The beginning – After welcoming people, the discussion lead should introduce the focus of the discussion and what will happen. The focus can be presented as an issue, such as sharing decision-making or promoting a positive culture, or as a question, for example 'Do we, the team here promote shared decision-making with patients/residents?' or 'Do we have a positive culture and how do we know?'

The middle – show or read the trigger/scenario and then pose a few open questions to get and keep the discussion going. For example:

- What are your initial feelings or thoughts about the . . . (DVD, factsheet, poster etc.)?
- Why do you feel or think that?
- What do you think was going on here?
- What are the key points that were being made?
- What are the key values being demonstrated?
- What is the . . . saying to you?
- Are there any similarities or differences with what happens in our care setting/home?
- Is there anything significant for us in this . . .?
- What can we learn from this . . .?
- Is there anything we wish to think further about in relation to the values we hold in our group or in the care setting/ home?
- Is there any action we want to take as a result of our discussion? If so, who is going to take that action, by when, who will they report back to and by when?

Avoid using closed questions which invite a straight Yes/No answer without an implicit invitation to explore the issue, for example 'Did the . . . (poster, video, scenario) make you feel sad?' or 'Do you agree that the key value here is that residents with dementia should be offered simple choices?' Also, avoid leading questions that point to the answer, for instance 'Is the main issue that comes out of the . . . (poster, video, scenario) that a resident is often not valued as a person by us as staff?' or 'Do you think that the key action is that we should ask patients/residents?

Summarise the key points of discussion, learning and action points on the flipchart paper as the discussion goes on. Point out the handout on 'How to feature values and beliefs in your work' for future reference.

The end – summarise the key points from the flipchart and emphasise the further thinking and/or action that may have been agreed. Ask people to evaluate the discussion honestly using one word. Chapter 8 is also useful in thinking about how to evaluate learning activities and to give and receive feedback in ways that help us to learn and not feel threatened.

Afterwards, store the notes/flipchart key points and actions to be taken safely as they can be used as evidence to describe where you are at the beginning of the journey to develop practice in your workplace, service or home.

Discussion trigger 2.1: Short videos

For ease of use, this trigger is also available on the companion website **www.wiley.com/go/practicedevelopment/ workbook**

If you have computer access for staff, patients and service users in your setting, you can use videos downloaded from the Internet. We have suggested a few websites below, as well as giving you some hints about finding your own triggers. There are a huge range of freely available videos in most health-care fields that you can choose from for your setting or care home. It is likely that you will be successful in finding videos that are relevant to your own profession or country.

The videos can be on very small 'screens', so if you have more than three or four group members coming to the discussion, you may need to invite them to view it before by setting it up somewhere accessible to them during the day or day before or at home.

You could start the discussion by asking people to share what stood out for them in the video or by following the suggestions on the Discussion Groups guidance.

Tip: Find a good trigger for your profession, field of practice and/or country.

To start surfing the Internet, google the following:

NHS patient stories

Patient experience videos

You could also access some of the websites listed in Chapter 1, for example the Picker Institute, the NHS Institute for Innovation and Improvement, or the Social Care Institute for Excellence (SCIE) to find material relevant to your setting/home.

Patient Stories   This is a social enterprise initiative that uses documentary and drama-documentary film-making techniques to provoke discussion and debate amongst health-care professionals about safety and quality issues (www.patientstories .org.uk).

Patients' Experiences   Patients with long-term conditions tell their stories about living with their conditions and how they cope (www.nhs.uk/Planners/Yourhealth/Pages/Realstories.aspx).

Institute for Healthcare Improvement
Hear our voice: collecting patient experience stories

Aims to engage health profession students in recording and analysing patient experience stories through which to highlight opportunities for local improvement and wider health-care reform (www.ihi.org/offerings/ihiopenschool/ resources/Pages/CollectingPatientExperienceStories.aspx).

Patient Voices: digital stories   The Patient Voices digital stories use video, audio, still images and music to convey patients', carers', practitioners' and managers' stories in a unique way. They are intended to help people to connect with lived experiences and motivate people working to improve the quality of health and social care (www.patientvoices.org.uk/stories.htm).

What do you see? film – YouTube   This arresting short film by Amanda Waring and starring Virginia McKenna is an excellent trigger for all health workers and professionals. It stimulates lasting conversations and deep reflection about person-centred care. It is based on the poem that you can read on the website (http://mrmom.amaonline.com/stories/Crabbit OldWoman.htm).

Social Care Institute for Excellence (SCIE)   (www.scie.org.uk/socialcaretv/topic.asp?guid=f616877d-62a1-4718-9c0e -f6a0ba1a7526)

For example, working with lesbian, gay, bisexual and transgendered people – older people and residential care: Roger's story (www.scie.org.uk/socialcaretv/video-player.asp?guid=CACAAE12-7375-429A-9D9A-1D28E29E65BD).

***My* home life**   Case studies are presented by short videos in the following areas:

- managing transitions;
- maintaining identity;

- creating community;
- sharing decision-making;
- improving health and health care;
- supporting good end-of-life;
- keeping workforce fit for purpose;
- promoting a positive culture.

(www.myhomelife.org.uk)

Dying Matters   The Dying Matters Coalition is working to address advance care planning by encouraging people to talk about their wishes towards the end of their lives, including where they want to die and their funeral plans with friends, family and loved ones. They've created a wide range of resources to help people start conversations about dying, death and bereavement. (www.dyingmatters.org/)

Hospice Friendly Hospitals   The work of the Hospice Friendly Hospitals (HFH) Programme is focused on making end-of-life care central to hospital care and on bringing it 'from the margins to the mainstream of health services'. The work of the programme is focused around four key themes: Competence & Compassion; Planning & Coordination; The Physical Environment; An Ethical Approach. Short video-clips (and other resources) to stimulate discussion of these themes are available online. (http://hospicefoundation.ie/what-we-do/hospice-friendly-hospitals/)

Sheets 2.4–2.8 set out a variety of further discussion triggers or activities you can use in your workplace and they can be found on the companion website (www.wiley.com/go/practicedevelopment/workbook).

Sheet 2.3: Handout: How to feature values and beliefs in your work around the care setting/care home

> *Handout for care setting/care home staff, leaders and managers*

The purpose of this handout is to provide you with some ideas about how to raise the profile of values and beliefs in your care setting/care home. This is important as a preparation for developing a shared vision in the workplace.

The handout includes ideas on:

- setting a *no blame* climate;
- showing how values and beliefs are influencing care and service in the setting/home;
- doing a quick evaluation to raise awareness of the values and beliefs team members say they have (ideal values) and the ones that actually drive care;
- pointing out and celebrating when there is a match between what people say their values are and the actual values seen in what they do.

Setting a no blame climate   In order to feature values and beliefs in your care setting/home, it is essential that a *no blame* climate is set and sustained. The reason for this is that when we become more aware of the actual values that are influencing the way we work with patients/residents, families and each other, the more aware we become that we might be falling short of our ideal values and beliefs. We might also begin to compare the actual values operating in the workplace with the values of being person-centred (see Chapter 1) and find them lacking.

The key thing that we need to accept is that it is part of being human not to always reach our ideals and live our values. We see this in our everyday lives, and even when we try really hard, we often fall short. The important thing is not to beat ourselves up, but to be constantly trying to reduce the gap between our ideal and actual values. For this to happen, we need to be open to feedback from others about the success or not of our attempts.

Reducing the gap and asking for, giving and receiving feedback and then using it constructively to learn requires self-awareness and emotional maturity. It also needs a climate or culture in which learning at work is an accepted way of life. Chapter 8 in this resource will be helpful here in creating a learning culture in your home. But for now, as you start your journey to develop practice by clarifying beliefs and values, try to respect the values that emerge especially if they are different from your own.

Showing how values and beliefs are influencing care and service in your setting/home   It is obvious that if you and your fellow workers are engaging in the learning activities in this chapter and the next, you will be raising the profile of values and beliefs. However, you can capitalise on this by building in opportunities to share the new insights about values and beliefs that are emerging. Opportunities include, for example, the shift handover – overlap time when early and late staff are working alongside each other – and any team or home meetings. Point out kindly when you see certain values in an interaction or intervention, in what someone says or doesn't say. Constantly remind yourself and others that when we expose our values to each other like this, we are going to honour and respect each other's values and beliefs. That we are not going to jump on each other like a ton of bricks or argue about who is right and who is wrong. Equally, point out where you see a good fit between the values that we say we use and the values that we actually use.

Quick evaluation   You might find that doing a quick evaluation and then discussing the results will alert team members to values and beliefs currently operating where they match or not with what we think they are. This discussion would be set in the context of an explicit intention to improve the experiences of patients and residents. The methods and tools presented in this chapter can help you with that. If you work in a care home, some simple questions, adapted from an AgeUK checklist, are provided for you at **www.wiley.com/go/practicedevelopment/workbook** that you might find helpful.

Celebrating a match between actual and person-centred values   When actual values match person-centred values, this is a cause for celebration. You can do this by pointing it out and saying 'well done' to your fellow worker or manager as you go about your everyday work. You might invite them to share that particular situation where the match occurred during the working day or in a discussion group. Simply saying 'well done' is enormously powerful in increasing a person's commitment to improving and developing practice.

Sheet 2.4: Values and beliefs template (Warfield & Manley 1990)

This tool is for individual use by care setting/care home staff, patients/residents, families, friends and volunteers. The topic to be explored is agreed by everyone.

I believe the ultimate purpose of _____ is:

I believe this purpose can be achieved by:

I believe the factors that help us achieve this purpose are:

I believe the factors that hinder us from achieving this purpose are:

Other values and beliefs I consider important in relation to _____ are:

Use the material you collect on here to take to a group discussion.

Sheet 2.5: Values and beliefs clarification activity: A facilitator's guide

> This guide is for the person who is facilitating the activity

This is a formal activity, starting off with individual work (as shown in the previous template), followed by group work. The group work is best facilitated by someone with facilitation skills.

The five questions to be answered by this exercise are:

1. What is the purpose of _____, for example person-centred care?
2. How can this purpose be achieved?
3. What are the factors that help us achieve this purpose?
4. What are the factors that hinder us in achieving this purpose?
5. What other values and beliefs do we hold in relation to _____, for example person-centred care?

Principles and things that you need to have before you start

- Get together a small group of four/five people to help you. If there is someone in your care setting/care home who has experience of analysing information, ask them to join you.
- Involve as many people as possible by inviting everyone in the care setting/care home to participate. You might do this by making an invitation (see Invitation and information sheet at **www.wiley.com/go/practicedevelopment/workbook** for a template that you can use) or poster and putting it on noticeboards or telling people and your fellow workers about it.
- Stress that it is really important for everyone to contribute openly and honestly because decisions will be made as a result of this activity.

You will need:

- a room to put up flipcharts for 3 weeks;
- five flipchart sheets with the instructions (see below) set out beside them;
- pens;
- sticky notes (five different colours).

You will need to stick the five flipchart sheets on the wall (see Figure 2.3). On the first sheet, put the first statement from the template at the top as a heading: for example, **I believe the purpose of person-centred** . . . .

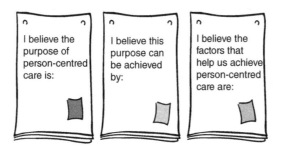

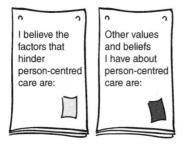

Fig. 2.3 Flipcharts with statements and coloured sticky notes.

care is . . . On the second sheet, put **I believe this purpose can be achieved by** . . . and so on. You may need more than one set of five sheets depending on the number of people you have. Choose five coloured sticky notes. Put a different colour sticky note securely on each flipchart sheet, beside the heading, so you have only one sticky note per heading.

The invitations: Setting out the purpose   It is important that you and the small group helping you set out the purpose of the activity briefly and clearly on the invitation and information sheet (see example at **www.wiley.com/go/ practicedevelopment/workbook**), poster or in conversations – something along these lines:

> This activity is to explore our values and beliefs about person-centred . . . . care. The purpose of the activity is to start developing shared values and beliefs about person-centred care. If we can develop and agree to a set of shared values and beliefs, we can become clearer about what we do and what we might want to do in regards to our care and service in this home. You are asked to contribute as much as you want and to do this as honestly as you can.

In conversations, ask people if they are clear about what you are inviting them to do and answer any questions they may have about the activity.

Instruction sheet   The instruction sheet (see **www.wiley.com/go/practicedevelopment/workbook** for a sample instruction sheet that you can use in your work) should be stuck on the wall beside the five flipchart sheets. Spare instruction sheets and numerous pads of sticky notes in the five colours (the five colours you have put on the flipcharts by the headings) should be placed nearby where everyone can see them.

Theming the statements   Once the data have been collected, the facilitator should gather and organise the data/feedback so that all the data about each statement are on the right flipchart sheets (this is why encouraging people to use the right colour sticky notes is so important in case some get detached by mistake; please refer to Figure 2.3). Theming of the statements should be a group exercise if possible involving patients/residents, families, visitors and team members. This can be a creative, learning exercise as well as part of work.

- The facilitator asks participants to organise themselves into small groups – one for each flipchart sheet/heading (thus if there are several flipchart sheets with the same heading on, a group will have only one stem or cue, but several flipchart sheets in front of them). Instruct them to read through the sticky notes and check out the meaning of the statements with each other. Then the groups should start to theme the notes on their flipchart sheets and give each theme a short name that accurately represents the content of that theme. The group chooses short phrases that describe that theme. These phrases are called attributes or characteristics. Look for patterns; for instance, you may see that some of the themes seem to link with each other. **Stress that themes, characteristics and patterns must be supported by what is written on the sticky notes, that is, no new ideas are brought in.**
- The exception for this process is the group who has the heading '*Other values and beliefs I consider important in relation to . . . .*'. They need to review the notes and see which of the other groups the notes can be given to. This requires a more in-depth knowledge about concepts of practice development, and may need the facilitator to support the group with reflective questions.
- Alternatively, the facilitator(s) can do this theming quickly and suggest which other flipcharts these other values and beliefs sticky notes could be added to.

Sharing the themes and drafting summary statements   Once the groups have achieved this, the facilitator asks each group to share their themes with the other groups. The facilitator again invites any focused comments on **what the themes mean**, as opposed to an open discussion about themes or whether they are 'correct'. (30 mins)

The facilitator invites comments from the participants on their experience of this activity and highlights any emergent learning points. At this point, each group and each stem/cue will have a set of themes and key elements or attributes. These are then transcribed onto a flipchart sheet.

Look at these two examples (and note the move from '<u>I</u> believe . . .' to '<u>We</u> believe . . .'):

Example 1 <u>We</u> believe the ultimate purpose of the oncology day-unit care is:

To keep patients safe (Theme 1 with five attributes):

- safe;
- good physical care;
- infection free;
- compliance with treatment regime;
- no complaints.

To feel confident in the team (Theme 2 with four attributes):

- to know who team members are;
- to know who will be caring for them;
- to express themselves;
- to have a choice and voice.

Example 2 <u>We</u> believe the ultimate purpose of dementia care is:
To keep patients/residents happy (Theme 1 with four attributes):

- safe;
- good physical care;
- calm;
- prevent challenging behaviours.

To feel emotionally safe (Theme 2 with four attributes):

- to take risks;
- to express themselves;
- to have choice and a sense of freedom;
- to feel listened to and valued.

The aim is to ask each group to write up a draft summary statement that captures concisely their theme and its attributes. This should not be done until the group have clarified what each concept and attribute means to them, especially if it is a piece of jargon or a buzz term. For example, you could ask: 'What do we mean by high standards?', 'What is sensitive care?' or 'Whose voice?' **Stress again that participants must only work with what they have and any connecting words that are needed, such as 'the', 'and', 'if', 'with' etc.**

Putting values and beliefs into practice   Once you have the four summary statements, you will need to help the group decide if others in the care setting/home not present need an opportunity to consider the draft values and beliefs and how this will happen. If a consultation is carried out, then you will have a set of shared values and beliefs that people **say** they have – but this is only the beginning. You now need to consider how to put these values and beliefs into practice. Two questions you can use to facilitate a discussion about this process are:

- How do you expect to see these shared values and beliefs used in the service offered to patients/residents and families?
- How do you expect gaps between these values and beliefs and the actual service given to be responded to?

This is about negotiating with team members, patients/residents and families about how the shared values and beliefs need to be a dynamic presence in practice, and what they can expect to happen if they are not used to shape practice, or, more importantly, where patients/residents and family experience does not match the stated values and beliefs.

This activity can also be carried out with families/friends.

NOTE
Relook at example 1:
To keep patients safe (Theme 1 with five attributes):

- safe;
- good physical care;
- infection free;
- compliance with treatment regime;
- no complaints.

   A facilitator would, for example, need to ask these team members what they would do if a patient declined certain treatment or wanted to make a complaint.
   Also relook at the second example from the care home team. How would team members respond when challenged by residents who took risks and expressed themselves and it potentially made them less safe?

Sheet 2.6: Instruction sheet for patients/residents, families and care staff for the values and beliefs clarification activity

This activity is to explore our values and beliefs about person-centred (*insert type of care*) . . . . care.

The purpose of the activity is to start developing shared values and beliefs about person-centred (*insert type of care*) . . . . care.

If we can develop and agree a set of shared values and beliefs, we can become clearer about what we do and what we might want to do in regards to our care and service.

You are asked to contribute as much as you want and to do this as honestly as you can.

- Please do this activity individually and do not talk with others about your values at this stage. This is because it is important that each of us can state what are really our own values and beliefs without being influenced by someone else.
- Take a few sticky notes in each of the five colours.
- You will see that each question on each flipchart has a different colour. For each flipchart statement, write as many different responses as you want to – but with only one response on each sticky note. Then put the notes on the flipchart sheets.
- Now have a look at what others have put on the flipchart sheets and add any further responses if you want to. Again, do this without talking to others. Please do not move anyone else's sticky note to another sheet and do not comment on what others have written.

This is also available on **www.wiley.com/go/practicedevelopment/workbook**

Chapter 3   Developing a Shared Vision for Person-Centred Care

Contents

Introduction

This chapter is adapted and then further redesigned from the work of the International Practice Development Collaborative (see Dewing & Titchen, 2007).[1]

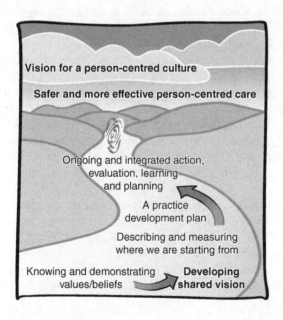

Fig. 3.1 The next step on the practice development journey: Developing a shared vision.

---

[1] The International Practice Development Collaborative (IPDC) is a community of practice (practice developers and researchers) who are committed to working together to develop healthcare practice. The IPDC believes that the aim of practice development is to work with people to develop person-centred cultures that are dignified, compassionate and safer for all. There are four pillars of work – Practice development schools; Online journal; Conferences; Symposia. The work of the IPDC is influenced and informed by the individual academic and scholarly work of the collaborators and practice partners. For information about the collaborators, please visit http://www.fons.org/library/about-ipdc.aspx

---

Practice Development Workbook for Nursing, Health and Social Care Teams, First Edition. Jan Dewing, Brendan McCormack, and Angie Titchen.
© 2014 John Wiley & Sons, Ltd. Published 2014 by John Wiley & Sons, Ltd.
Companion website: www.wiley.com/go/practicedevelopment/workbook

> At the end of Chapter 2, your team may have clarified its values and beliefs. If you have, you will have arrived at four summary statements about the values you hold in relation to person-centred care. By being involved in the activities set out in Chapter 3, everyone in the team can have the opportunity to build on those summary statements to develop a shared vision in the form of a written statement. The variety of activities here offers you choice in how you might do this work together.
>
> Chapter 3 also offers guidance to those team members who may be beginning to take a lead in developing practice. The guidance here is about setting up a coordinating group and the kind of activities the lead person might offer everyone in the team, whatever care setting you work in.

What is a shared vision?

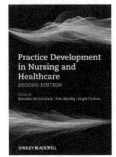

At its simplest, a shared vision answers the question 'What do we want to create?' In developing practice or 'practice development', this is often described as your 'ultimate purpose'. A shared vision is not just a collection of words; it represents the values team members, patients, residents, families, carers, service managers, executives and board members carry in both their heads and their hearts. A shared vision is what people want to move towards. You might like to read Chapter 3 in McCormack et al. (2013) for an example of how a shared vision is central to a whole organisational approach to practice development.

A vision is shared when two or more people have a similar image or mental picture of what they want to create and commit to with one another to make it happen.

> Consider for a moment if you went around your care setting and described to others your vision for how the place could be in three years' time. How long would it take until someone said 'That's exactly the way I see it too?'

The greater the involvement of all team members in creating the vision, the more powerful the vision can become. Thus the processes used to help create the shared vision are crucial. In the course of our practice development work, we have found that a strong bond and sense of purpose is created when the team share a common vision that they have created rather than one they are given.

Most team members, like most people, want to be a part of something bigger, and a shared vision provides that. Shared vision is vital in order for teams, services and indeed, for whole organisations to succeed. This is because it provides a focus and creates energy for 'new' work. Where there is no shared vision, teams might talk about a lack of direction or of feeling as though they are drifting. They lose trust in those they feel should be helping to provide vision.

In developing practice, we all have a responsibility for developing the vision, not just a select few. Unlike many leadership theories, practice development stresses that the shared vision is developed by everyone rather than it being the leader's vision that is adopted. Without a shared vision, separate self-interests can override collaborative interests. However, a shared vision should still help reasonable personal visions to be achieved, and reasonable individual needs to be met.

As well as providing a focal point for the future, a shared vision is a base from which you can evaluate your current practices and the culture in the care setting or care home. It helps you to make decisions about how suggested new ways of working will contribute to the shared vision. Thus, the vision statement can be used as part of everyday practice development work. It can and needs to be made real in several ways.

For example: asking the team to reflect on current practice against the shared vision; using the vision to help team members to visualise the journey to achieving it and what it would feel like to be living the vision; through the use of certain *challenging* questions.

General examples:

> 'Let's talk about how (*insert description of current practice*) fits with our vision for a quality rapid discharge service.'
>
> 'Let's think about how (*insert description of current practice*) fits with our vision for a quality pre-operative admission nursing led assessment service.'
>
> 'Let's examine how (*insert description of current practice*) fits with our vision for a quality care home.'

Specific examples:

> 'Let's talk about how carrying out intentional care rounds contributes to our vision for a patient-centred and safer service where patients and families know what is happening.'

'Let's consider how enabling choice about what time to take medication in the morning fits with our vision for a person-centred service.'

'Let's explore how not giving people choice about what time they get up in the morning fits with our vision for a person-centred service.'

'Let's think about how our reservations about having a residents' group fits with our vision for involvement in the running of the care home.'

'How does enabling patients to write in their care records fit with our vision?'

Shared visions emerge from personal visions and personal visions emerge from values and beliefs (see Chapter 2). Expression of personal values and beliefs is thus central to successfully contributing to a collaborative vision within your team. Depending on the team and people you are working with, and the time you have for this work, you may need to do some preparatory work to help people to talk about their personal visions (based on their own values and beliefs). However, it is possible to undertake values and beliefs work and then move straight into shared vision work all together.

Weaving in elements of the background information offered in this introduction, as you introduce and facilitate vision work, may assist groups to make more sense of the purpose of developing a shared vision. Where people in the team have different cultural experiences, language skills and ways of understanding, you might need to explain what a shared vision is in words and ways they can understand (which might include pictures, for example).

Once a shared vision has been created and then agreed, it is important that you facilitate a discussion about the expectations of what needs to happen to ensure the vision becomes a part of practice, using a key question such as:

'How will we help each other to work to our shared vision?' or

'How will we make use of this shared vision in our everyday practice?'

Resources in this chapter

- **Setting up a coordinating group** – when beginning to think about building on the activities in Chapter 2 (identifying and sharing values and beliefs about care) for creating a shared vision, it is a good idea to think about how visioning activities can be coordinated and sustained in the team. In the guide here, we offer some ideas about setting up and running a coordinating group that works in person-centred ways.

   Group relaxation activity – you can find this resource on the website **www.wiley.com/go/practicedevelopment/ workbook**. This is a warm-up activity and can be used to enable a relaxed and creative atmosphere in a group – just what is needed for creative vision work.

- **Creative methods for developing a shared vision** – in this chapter we have set out various methods, i.e. workshops, visioning with a virtual group and a questionnaire for developing a shared vision. As the workshops are similar in some ways, we offer you a programme, which briefly sets out the differences, to help you choose the workshop that will suit you, your team and workplace best. Whatever method you choose to use, we encourage you to use the method more or less as we have set it out before you amend it. This is just so you can be confident and competent in delivering the core stages of the method before adding your own touches or becoming more adventurous.

   Introducing creativity helps balance left brain activity (rational, analytical thinking) with right brain activity (creative imagination) and is more likely to release greater potential and achieve a fuller range of options. Three of the workshops incorporate creative methods, along with a more formal values clarification activity. Bringing in creative methods helps us to use our imaginations and creativity to build a vision for person-centred care. They can also be more fun!

   Some team members may have creative hobbies and use creative arts, but for many working with creativity, especially at work, is a new experience. We have found that people experience a variety of feelings in response to the prospect of exploring the use of their creative imagination. These feelings may include shyness, embarrassment, anxiety, excitement and pleasure. These are all natural and usual responses to new ways of learning and engaging in learning. It is vital that a facilitator creates a safe and open space in which everyone who takes part can explore and learn in new ways.

   We suggest that you may find it useful to encourage people to reflect on how they feel about participating in a workshop with creative methods, and to think about the kinds of support strategies they would find helpful. In our experience, feedback on creative methods included comments such as: 'sceptical and then sold', 'felt a bit vulnerable/

self-conscious, but see its potential value', 'very good, more of this type of work would be useful', 'amazed at its power', 'great opportunity to see and experience visioning'.

Before using these various methods in creating a shared vision, it is necessary that shared values and beliefs have been established (see Chapter 2). This can be done some time before the vision work, or in the first part of a longer group or workshop event. For *Vision statement development*, the facilitator will need draft summary statements like those we describe being created in Chapter 2. Creative materials will be required for *Visualisation through painting and/or collage*.

- **Visioning the practice development processes and developing ground rules** – these one-to-one, small informal group and formal workshop resources can be used to ensure that the *processes* for how the vision will be achieved are discussed. These processes must be consistent with the values and beliefs, for example, of being person-centred. This activity can often form a bridge into the more structured and practical activity of writing a practice development plan. This activity needs creative materials, plus photos, pictures or postcards – full details are given in the resource. You will also need draft summary statements like those we describe being created in Chapter 2.
- **What do we do next?** – the chapter closes by explaining what you will be doing with the shared vision now that it has been developed, i.e. how you will use it to design your baseline (starting point) evaluation and then, once the evaluation is done, create the practice development plan for your service or care home. Whilst these activities will take some time, we also suggest things that you can begin to do straight away.

Guide: Setting up a practice development coordinating group for visioning activities

This guide is for those who are beginning to take a lead in developing practice in the care setting or care home

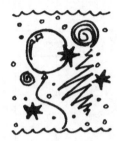

Whoever is initiating this group needs to work in partnership with the formal leader of the service (such as unit manager or home/ward manager) to identify up to six people who you think would be willing and able to undertake this work and who also reflect the diversity or spread of everyone who works in the team as much as possible. Finding out who has enjoyed and undertaken activities in Chapter 2 of this resource might help you to identify potential group members. In the setting-up phase, it is important to be very clear for yourself, potential group members and everyone in the team, that the purpose of the group is merely to kick start the practice development journey by coordinating the visioning work and trying to do that in person-centred ways. It should also be made clear that an overarching practice development coordinating group will eventually be needed but that the purpose, role and membership of that group will be guided by the vision that is created by all stakeholders.

The first task of the coordinating group might be to look at the activities in this chapter and establish whether there is anyone in the wider service or care home who has the skills to facilitate the workshops and activities. Think widely, if no one immediately springs to mind, there may be a volunteer or a team member such as the chaplain that has experience of working with small groups. If no one comes to mind, then talk with someone more senior or someone who works in Learning and Development or the service manager about getting outside support to help you to provide the activities, so that things get off to a good start. The skills of helping members in small groups to work together (in person-centred ways) will come in very handy on your practice development journey to person-centred care. **If you cannot find such help and there is no one in your organisation with such experience, we suggest that you use the group relaxation activity, followed by the vision statement development workshop, as this combination is the simplest and it is building on the values clarification activity in Chapter 2.**

It is likely that your group will need to coordinate a number of repeat activities to ensure that everyone has the opportunity to contribute to the visioning activity if they want to. So you will need to plan when, where and how often and who is responsible for what. For example, you may decide that one person will be responsible for creating posters explaining the visioning activity and inviting people to attend (including the time and place).

Other responsibilities might include:

- explaining to as many people as possible why the team is creating a shared vision and how it is going about it;
- getting materials for the workshops;
- if there have been separate activities, making sure that all the shared vision statements are collected together and stored carefully;
- deciding who will put all the statements together to write joint statements and how the joint statements will be circulated for comment;
- how comments and views on the joint statements will be fed back and to whom and what will happen next;
- how the shared vision will be launched and celebrated.

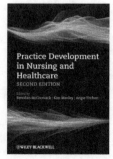

At this stage, it may be useful for the group to look at the Frequently Asked Questions, in Chapter 9, in relation to the questions relevant to 'When you start working on developing a shared vision for person-centred care'. You may also find using the following templates makes the meetings of the coordinating group as efficient and democratic as possible. Finally, you might find it useful to read Chapter 8 of McCormack et al. (2013); in particular, we would recommend you read story 8.3 in that chapter. This story illustrates how a facilitator leads a group through a visioning process with a focus on the safeguarding of vulnerable adults in a hospital setting – the processes can be applied to any setting, however.

Sheet 3.1: Templates for group meeting agendas and notes

Visioning Coordination Group Session

AGENDA

Date: _____ Time: _____ Place: _____
Facilitator: _____
Note-taker: (to record briefly decisions and actions) _____

Agenda item	What is to be decided/agreed/actioned	Who will present item

Date: _____

NOTES

Agenda item	Decisions/agreements/ actions	Person responsible	By when	Progress

Sheet 3.2: Group relaxation activity

This activity aims to clear the head and create a more relaxed feeling in a group in readiness for creative visioning work. It is provided for you on **www.wiley.com/go/practicedevelopment/workbook**

This relaxation activity, or a similar one, is carried out at the beginning of the workshop or event where developing a shared vision is taking place. If you are combining a values and beliefs exercise with vision development, then the relaxation can be done at the very start.

Sheet 3.3: Creative methods for developing a shared vision: Programme of three workshops (you decide which one you might do)

Guide for a new facilitator

These workshops provide opportunities for new facilitators to work in person-centred ways with small groups. The workshops link with the values clarification method described in Chapter 2. Participants will build on the work they have done to clarify their own values and beliefs and use it to build a vision together. Participants will practise a key skill of being person-centred – the capacity to accept that others may have different values, experiences and views to theirs. They will be able to practise listening attentively to others and not being judgemental or trying to interpret the other people's expressions of their visions.

Visualisation through painting and/or collage

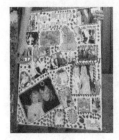

In this one and a half hour workshop, people will be invited to create a painting or collage that reflects their vision and aspirations of their practice and workplace. It is based on the idea that creating something helps us to understand what the future might look like, and it can also help us to begin to open up talking about what needs to happen to make the vision real. There will be a conversation about what emerges. You will have the opportunity to practise using creativity as a means of bringing up values that are so much a part of us that they are difficult to talk about.

Visioning

This creative workshop is shorter and can be done in 30–45 minutes, so if time is tight, then you may choose this option. Through creative visualisation, the facilitator takes people on an imaginary journey through which they explore whatever comes spontaneously into their imagination, using all the senses (imaginatively). You will have the chance to stretch your mind and open up to new ways of doing things.

Vision statement development

Whilst vision work is always going to involve an element of imagination about what might and could be, some people may find it difficult to engage in the creative approaches above. Thus, this 1 hour workshop may be more suitable for people who prefer to work through analysis and discussion. In this workshop, a vision statement can be generated from the summary of the values and beliefs work (see Chapter 2). You will be able to practise involving everyone in reaching agreement. However, doing a group relaxation activity first might be a gentle introduction to more imaginative approaches for these people (**www.wiley.com/go/practicedevelopment/workbook**).

Sheet 3.4: Workshop guidance: Visualisation through painting and/or collage

Guide for a new facilitator

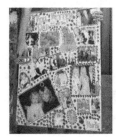

This group activity would give a new facilitator a chance to practise helping people in a small group (maximum of eight) to work together effectively. If possible, the new facilitator could also work alongside a more experienced facilitator for a group of 20–25.

The aim of this workshop is for a small group of people, such as team members, clinical leaders or team leaders in the care setting or across the patient pathway to develop a shared personal vision for the future that will guide the practice development work. Depending on your service, you may also want to include patients/residents, families, carers and volunteers.

People will be invited to create a painting or collage that reflects their vision and aspirations of their practice and workplace. Creating something generates understanding about what the future is going to look like and people can begin to open up, talking about what needs to happen to make the vision real.

You will need:

- 1.5 hours;
- a large room with chairs around the side and some tables for those who want to work on a surface;
- one or two facilitators (usually two facilitators for 20–25 participants);
- materials for painting; felt-tip pens, crayons, pastels (plus any other drawing materials you want to include); newspaper or other floor covering if paint is being used;
- materials for collage include the above plus magazines and newspapers or a supply of images; clay, scissors, glue sticks; everyday small leftover and 'junk' items (e.g. wine bottle tops/corks, plastic containers), leaves, flowers, small twigs and branches, silver-coloured foil, coloured paper, tissue papers and card, felt;
- a flipchart easel, paper and marker pens.

Key activities

Introduction and purpose of workshop. (5 mins)

Creative work individually in a quiet or silent space. (15 mins)

Ask participants to organise themselves into small groups where each individual shares the meaning of their painting or collage and the group records on flipchart sheets the key attributes of each personal vision. (15 mins)

Open gallery viewing and sharing of paintings and collages and the creator's intended message. (15 mins)

If you have longer and want to include a discussion at this point, you can achieve this by inviting responses on the work based on the following:

- I see . . .
- I feel . . .
- I imagine . . .

Do not encourage discussion about the 'artistic' quality of the work or viewers telling the creator of the work what the work means.

Discussion in the large group or several smaller groups based on the key questions (45 mins):

- What is our shared vision for future practice and our ward, unit, care home or service?
- What are the key features of future practice and our ward, unit, care home or service?
- How will we move towards our new vision?

Summarise the purpose of the work and the emerging points and suggest that participants consider what they have learned from the creative method. Outline what will happen next to build on the collaborative work.

Close.

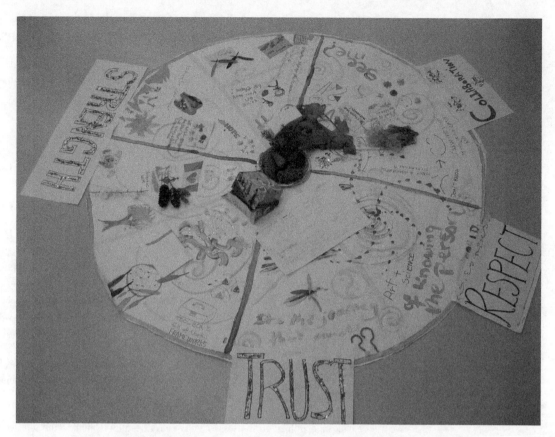

Fig. 3.2 An example of using painting and collage in practice development work.

Note the team's clarified values and beliefs positioned around the edge of the circle.

Sheet 3.5: Workshop guidance: Creating and sharing personal visions

Guide for an experienced facilitator

This workshop can be offered to team members and other stakeholders by an experienced facilitator. If possible, a novice facilitator could experience the visualisation as a participant and then work alongside the experienced facilitator by writing on the flipchart for example.

The aim of this workshop is to develop and share personal visions with patients/residents and staff in the service setting or care home.

Time   30–45 minutes

First create a space in the room, pushing back tables and chairs if necessary. Invite people to make themselves comfortable, on a chair or on the floor. You might like to put something in the centre, on the floor, for example a jug of flowers or leaves and a candle and play some gentle music. The space is now ready for the visioning exercise.

Explain that the purpose of this session is to help people to use their creative imagination to create their own personal vision for their ward, unit, department or care home in the future. Visioning in this way helps us to tap into stuff that is usually difficult to talk about, either because there are no words for it or because it is so deeply ingrained in us that we take it for granted and don't normally talk about it.

The overall method is to take people on a journey in which they explore whatever comes into their imagination, using all the senses (imaginatively). It is important not to get in the way of people's imagination, so the facilitator might say something like this:

> We will be imagining with all our senses, where we have been (in relation to the service we work in and people we have worked with (or who have looked after us), where we would like our care and service to go and how we could get there. It is really important on this journey that you participate in a way that feels right for you. Please do not push yourself to follow my suggestions if they don't feel right. Do your own thing. Also, try to go with whatever comes into your imagination, however bizarre, and do not try to analyse it away. Our imagination often holds just the right message for us . . .

Begin with an exercise that helps people to become grounded. This often involves closing our eyes (except the facilitator) and becoming aware of our own breathing. For example:

> 'I suggest that we start with a grounding exercise, which will help us to let go of our busyness or whatever we have been doing and come into the 'here and now' and be truly present. Close your eyes now and listen to the sounds outside the room. We are going to leave the outside world for a time, letting go, for now, our thoughts about all our responsibilities at work and at home and our hopes, fears and expectations for this visioning session. Bring your attention to the sounds inside this room (pause). . . . And now, to the sounds within yourself. Listen to your breath (pause) and feeling the rise and fall of the chest (pause). . . . Letting go as we breathe out . . .' pause.

Then help people into an imaginary scene, for example a country landscape, beside the sea, up in the sky, a city dwelling – whatever, using any of a number of devices, such as going down through the earth by following the roots of a tree or going up to the sky by following the branches or walking across different kinds of ground. Invite people to choose a way in that is right and feels safe for them (say, e.g. 'If you don't want to go through the earth, you might like to set out on an imaginary walk across a muddy field, along a beach or in a city'. Thus we are sensitive to those who might feel fears such as claustrophobia or who have a fear of heights). Encourage people to accept the scene that opens up before them.

Exploration of the past, future and present by going to the place in the scene that represents what it was like to give or receive care/services in the care home in the past, the future and the present. Invite participants to journey back to that past. When they get there suggest they move, in their imagination, around their past. Ask them:

What do you:

- see?
- hear?
- taste?

- smell?
- feel (touch and emotions)?

After what feels like an appropriate amount of quiet or silence, invite participants to start moving towards their future in the service or care home in any way that springs from their imagination. Suggest they notice what they see, hear, smell, taste and feel on this part of the journey. When they arrive at their future, ask participants to really focus on noticing as much as they can and taking notice of their emotions. After a while, suggest they look back over their shoulder at where they have come from in their past. After a period of quiet or silence invite participants to set off back to the present and the care/services that is/are given and received in the care home/service (ward, unit etc.) today and then to explore it and imagine how they would get from this to the care/services of the future.

Bring people back to the actual present, into the room, by retracing their steps, for example helping them come back through the earth or along the branches back to the base of the tree or whatever. Give people time. When they emerge, you might say:

> When you are ready, gently open your eyes. If you would like to, pair up for a few minutes with someone near you and share your experience of past, future, present and how you made the journey from present to future. Or, you may prefer to spend the time alone and make a few notes or a drawing of what you have experienced.

Then invite sharing in the larger group about what they imagined and/or about the experience of visioning. The facilitator then asks participants to think about their experience and how this can be related to the way the team currently work with people. This part of the work can be carried out through small group discussion and using flipchart recordings to capture the vision statement and its features and how it is different from what happens now.

Examples

Martin, an assistant practitioner working across nursing and therapies in the community talked about how he heard a lot of crackling paper – as if it was dried out and crispy. He couldn't really see anyone's faces and no one talked to him. People all looked miserable and unhappy even in their own homes. He said he felt powerless, that although he wanted to change things he couldn't. When the facilitator asked Martin how he saw the future for his community rehabilitation based service, he went on to say that he saw everyone with a face and a name and he heard conversations and laughter going on. These conversations were not just about rehabilitation, he said, but about other things that mattered to the service users. Martin commented that this activity helped him to realise that the team might be too focused on their tasks rather than on building relationships with service users.

During a group session in a care home, Ella, a volunteer who had been working in the home for 20 years, described how when she went back to the past, she saw grey uniformity. She could smell and taste soggy cabbage and hear only chaotic shouting or screaming. The surfaces she could feel were hard and featureless. She thought that this linked with the institutionalised care that people with dementia had received in the care home long ago and showed the hopelessness felt by many older people and staff alike. She felt that although the fabric of the care home had improved over the last 10 years, the sense of hopelessness was still very strong.

She described the future as a rainbow, full of colour and embracing differences. She could smell freshly baked apple pie with cinnamon and could feel her taste buds responding. She could hear music and voices talking together. She could feel different textures – soft fabrics, wood, smooth stones, water and fresh grass. This reflected how she felt that the environment of the care home could be enriched by having more textures and plants in the home and improving access into the garden for residents. She had also read about residents organising baking sessions in their care home and described a photo of a woman with dementia doing a cookery demonstration.

The group were really taken by how quite simple actions could radically change things and discussed the idea that maybe their vision statement should include people with dementia sharing decision-making about the home environment and activities.

Whilst some participants report they get a lot out of this method, others say it does very little or even nothing for them. So, you will need to have a repertoire of methods for visioning and to know when the time is right to bring in any of the creative imagination methods. At the same time, gentle encouragement of participants to use their creative imagination in visioning work offers new learning experiences for stretching the mind and trying something new. It's vital to bring the imaginative element back to what this means for your care setting and the way care is organised and delivered.

Sheet 3.6: Workshop guidance: Vision statement development

Guide for a new facilitator

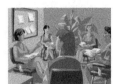

This workshop can be run by new facilitators who have experienced the values clarification method in Chapter 2 as some of the processes are similar. It is suggested that you/they seek support from someone with more experience of facilitation to help them prepare.

The aim of this method is to generate a shared vision statement about person-centred care that sets out the aspirations for the practice development. The processes of the workshop itself will help you to learn how to be democratic and person-centred in the ways that you work together in your workplace. In other words, that everyone has a voice in creating and agreeing the vision statement.

Vision work involves an element of imagination about what might and can be. Thus the creative methods set out above enable creativity to come to the fore. If this is felt inappropriate for any reason, a vision statement can be generated from the summary of the values and beliefs work (see Chapter 2).

A vision statement comprises a summary of:

- the ultimate purpose of . . . . (e.g. our work, our ward, our service, our care home, person-centred care);
- how that purpose can best be achieved;
- what factors will help with the achievement of the shared vision.

You will need:

- 1 hour;
- a large room with chairs well spaced out;
- one or two facilitators (usually two facilitators to 20–25 participants);
- a flipchart easel, paper and marker pens;
- flipchart sheets with the sticky notes that captured the themes from a values and beliefs clarification and the draft summary statements (see Values and beliefs clarification method in Chapter 2).

The participants are divided into three groups and the facilitator provides cues and instructions for the activity. Each group takes one of the draft summary statements from the values and beliefs work and ensures that there is a coherent summary statement written that captures the themes generated from the values and beliefs clarification. (15 mins)

The groups identify any jargon or confusing terminology in the statement and debate the possible meanings of the terms until agreement is reached. (20 mins)

Each group then shares the terminology that was under debate and the proposed agreed meanings. The other groups have an opportunity to question or add further debate until agreement is reached. The facilitator's focus is to promote open discussion and guide the groups to reach agreement. (20 mins)

Summary statements may need to be rewritten depending on the outcome of the group work. Any key points needed for clarification of terms are captured on flipchart sheets. The facilitator summarises the session, or asks the participants to summarise the session, and identifies individual learning and its relationship to developing practice. Action points for the next steps can be negotiated. The key aspects of this session are to promote an active debate on taken-for-granted jargon or confusing terms to ensure that the group has a shared understanding of meanings. This helps with clarity in the vision work and also enables participants to be more confident when talking about the vision to others.

Sheet 3.7: Guide: Visioning with a virtual group

Guide for a beginning facilitator

It is important that everyone in the care setting or care home has the opportunity to contribute to the visioning activity. This is because everyone needs to feel that their voice is heard, so they can really own and share the vision. However, it is not always possible for everyone to attend workshops together due to all the usual things of shift patterns, part-time work, a prior engagement and so on. Therefore, think ahead when you are planning a workshop or group event, about how you can provide an opportunity for those who are unable to attend to have their say. If you do this in advance, then you can feed in what they say at the event. Or you could do it the other way around. So, for example, after the event, send the summary vision statements and ideas that came out to those who could not attend and ask them for their responses and contributions. This opportunity could also be built into the questionnaire in the next resource.

> You could write out each summary statement followed by a Yes/No box to indicate agreement or not and a 'Please comment and add any of your own ideas in the space below'.

Another idea is that you invite contributions in a similar form to the one used at the event. Contributions might be paintings or collages of the vision as they see it, as in the example below, or a visualisation as shown in the questionnaire in the next resource.

Example

A ward team caring for patients with rheumatology were coordinating the vision development for the ward. Current in-patients had already contributed but because many patients were frequently re-admitted to the ward, they decided to offer such people an opportunity to contribute to the vision at the out-patient clinics over a 3-week period. Therefore, in collaboration with the outpatient staff, they covered a wall in the outpatient waiting area with flipchart paper stuck together with sticky tape on the back. The outpatient staff agreed to invite patients who had been looked after on the ward previously to contribute to a visual image of the vision. They set out paints and collage material and a waterproof table covering. They invited people to use the materials to create a representation of the ward as they would like it to be, should they be re-admitted in the future. Sticky notes were also provided for people to post comments about what they felt, saw and imagined when they looked at the whole collage/painting that was emerging.

If your group were using this approach in a longer-term in-patient or residential setting, you could invite a few representatives who had contributed to the visual image to look at it and respond to the emerging vision. Your group would capture these responses and feed them into the vision development done in the workshops when the summary statements were being put together.

Sheet 3.8: Questionnaire: Developing a shared vision for person-centred care at
. . . .

Dear _____

It is very important that everyone working in _____ has the opportunity to contribute to the visioning activity. This is because everyone in the team and connected to it needs to feel that their voice is heard, so they can really own and share the vision that is created. As you may know, the team has been offering several activities to give people this opportunity but there are some of us who have been unable to attend. Therefore, we are offering you a chance now to contribute your ideas and visions on how person-centred care could be in our care setting in the future.

In the activities, people used creative approaches to help them imagine the possible futures, as well as sharing ideas and talking about them. We offer you that chance too in this brief questionnaire in a modified form to take an imaginary journey into the past, future and present. You might want to read the following instructions and then close your eyes and go into your imagination.

Think back now to an aspect of your care in the past. Move around it in your imagination. Give yourself time.
What does that past look/smell/feel/sound/taste like?

_____

Now imagine care in the future here at _____. Move around it in your imagination.

_____

What does that future look/smell/feel/sound/taste like?

_____

Now come back to the present at your care setting. Move around it in your imagination.

What does the present look/smell/feel/sound/taste like?

_____
_____
_____

And what does the path to the future look/smell/feel/sound/taste like?

_____
_____
_____

What obstacles or barriers do you feel are present?

_____
_____
_____

Please complete and return this questionnaire to:

_____

Thank you

Sheet 3.9: Visioning the practice development processes and developing ground rules (one-to-one)

Guide for anyone working in any care setting

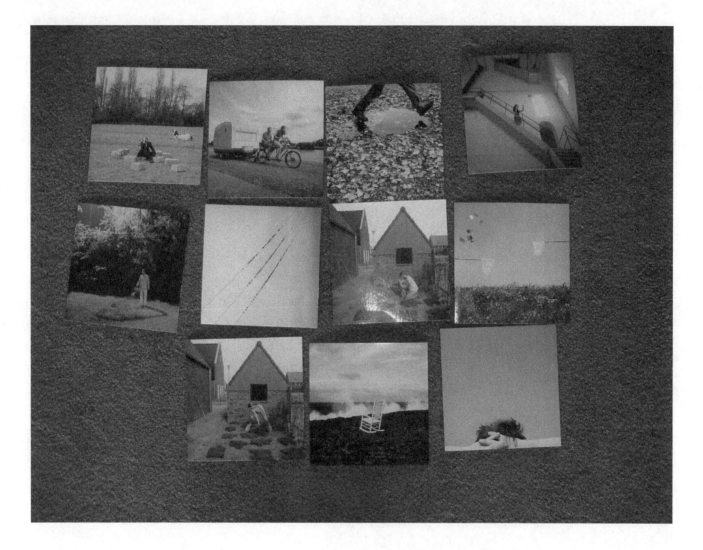

After the shared vision is agreed, you can do this activity with your learning buddy, clinical supervisor or person of your choosing or with any work groups you get involved in to begin to explore how to put the vision into action. The purpose of this activity is to generate shared ideas about the processes that you can use (and are preferable to use) so that the shared values and beliefs are lived and the vision is helped to become a reality. For example, a process would be *respecting* and *listening* to others' views without interruption. Another example is *getting to know* patients, service users or residents as people with unique hopes, likes, dislikes, fears and expectations. A practical outcome is the generation of ground-rules or a contract for learning together.

You will need:

- 30 minutes;
- a set of cards (you may have got a set if you did the first activity in Chapter 2 – if not have a look there for ideas of how to get or collect a set).
- a couple of pieces of flipchart paper and pens;
- summary of values and beliefs statements, including the enabling and hindering factors.

Key activities

Lay out the cards face up on the floor, ground or table. Then sit quietly for a moment, giving yourself a moment to make a clear break from the work you have just been doing. Take a few deep breaths and relax as you breathe out. Then choose the cards (as many as you want) that attract you – you don't have to have any reason at all, at this point, other than that you notice them above the others. (3 mins)

Now separately lay out the cards you have chosen, and really look at them. Ask yourself these questions and write a few notes if you wish: (5 mins)

- What do I like about this card(s) and why?
- Look at the summary values and beliefs statements, then back at your cards; does anything about the card symbolise or represent a process that would help you to live up to the values in the summary statements in your learning relationship with each other?
- What else does the card say about the ways you could work together on on the practice development journey?

Share your responses with each other and write up the processes you agree on the flipchart paper.

Discuss whether these are processes that you want to sign up to with your buddy. Check if there are any other processes that would be important to you both in your work together, and if there are, add them to your agreed list.

You have now got a set of agreed ground rules or principles for engagement for your partnership!

Consider whether you should do a similar activity with others in your care setting, perhaps those in the team you work with or, if you are a patient/resident, with other patients/residents who are setting up a working group to organise something. If you think it would be helpful, then you could suggest the next activity to the team or group.

You might like to add your ground rules or contract for learning together onto the worksheet we introduced in Chapter 1.

Example of ground rules

Respect each other as a person and co-worker and the different values, beliefs and views you each may hold.

Listen to each other actively and do not talk over each other.

Offer each other high challenge and high support.

Give each other feedback as a learning opportunity.

Receive feedback non-defensively.

Maintain confidentiality about what you tell each other unless you each agree otherwise.

However, if it is important for the practice development to share what you have discussed, agree that anonymised information can be shared with others (of course, you are free to share your own experiences with anyone you choose as they belong to you).

Carry out the actions you agree/commit to.

You can make up your own picture/word card packs or buy packs from several sources. One such resource is Evoke cards. Available from: http://www.evokecards.com/

Sheet 3.10: Visioning the practice development processes and developing ground rules (small informal group)

Guide for a new facilitator

This group activity would give a novice facilitator a chance to practise helping people in a small group to work together effectively.

After the shared vision is agreed, you can do this activity to begin to explore how to put the vision into action with your team or any small practice development groups that are being set up in the care setting or home.

The purpose of this activity is to generate shared ideas about the processes that you can use (and are preferable to use) so that the shared values and beliefs are lived and the vision is helped to become a reality. For example, a process would be helping everyone in the group to be included, work together and *clarifying* and *negotiating* roles and responsibilities in the group. A practical outcome of this activity is the generation of ground rules or principles for ways of working together as a group.

You will need:

- 30 minutes;
- you taking the role and responsibility of facilitator (see Chapter 8);
- a set of cards (perhaps you or one of the group has got a set now if you/they did the first activity in Chapter 2 – if not, have a look there for ideas of how to get or collect a set);
- a flipchart easel, paper and pens;
- summary of values and beliefs statements, including the enabling and hindering factors.

Key activities

Lay out the cards face up on the floor, ground or table. Then invite the group to sit quietly for a moment, giving themselves a moment to make a clear break from the work they have just been doing. Suggest they take a few deep breaths and relax as they breathe out. Then choose the cards (as many as they want) that attract them. Say that they don't have to have any reason at all for picking them, at this point, other than that they are drawn to them above the others. (3 mins)

Now invite people to separately lay out the cards they have chosen and really look at them. Invite them to ask themselves the following questions and write a few notes if they wish: (5 mins)

- What do I like about this card(s) and why?
- Look at the summary values and beliefs statements, then back at your cards; does anything about the card symbolise or represent a process that would help you to live up to the values in the summary statements in your working relationship with the group?
- What else does the card say about the ways you could work together on the practice development journey?

Ask them to share their responses and then discuss whether they agree with each other about them or not. You write up the processes they can all agree on on the flipchart.

Encourage discussion on whether these processes are ones that the group wants to sign up to as ground rules or principles for ways of working. Check if there are any other processes that would be important to them in their work together and if there are, add them to the agreed list.

The group now has a set of agreed ground rules or principles for ways of working together.

Example of ground rules

Respect each other as people and co-workers and the different values, beliefs and views you all may hold.

Listen to each other actively and do not talk over each other.

Don't blame each other or others for when things go wrong, but look for why they went wrong and plan together how to put them right.

Offer each other high challenge and high support.

Give each other honest feedback as a learning opportunity.

Receive feedback non-defensively.

Maintain confidentiality about what you tell each other unless you each agree otherwise.

However, if it is important for the practice development to share what you have discussed, agree that anonymised information can be shared with others (of course, you are free to share your own experiences with anyone you choose as they belong to you).

Carry out the actions you agree/commit to.

Share out the responsibilities the group takes on in the future, for example take turns with organising meetings, taking notes, or sharing the actions to be carried out.

Sheet 3.11: Workshop guidance: Visioning the practice development processes and developing ground rules

Guide for an experienced facilitator

This workshop can be run by experienced facilitators for a larger number of people.

After the shared vision is agreed, this workshop can be run at a different time to begin to explore how to put the vision into action. The purpose of the creative method in this workshop is to generate shared ideas about the processes that can be used and are preferable to use so that the shared values and beliefs are lived and the vision is being enabled. A practical outcome is the generation of ground rules or a contract for working together (see example in previous activity).

You will need:

- 1–2 hours (or longer depending on the size of the group);
- a large room with chairs well spaced out;
- one or two facilitators (usually two facilitators to 20–25 participants);
- a flipchart easel, paper and marker pens;
- photos or pictures/postcards of as many images of objects in the natural and 'man'-made world as possible, such as flowers, trees, birds, the ocean, waves, shells, cars, computers, maps, roads, foods, sweets, books, abstract paintings and so on;
- magazines, paper, pens, paints and brushes;
- summary of values and beliefs statements, including the enabling and hindering factors, somewhere where everyone can see them.

This activity can be done with large numbers of people working in small groups or with a small group working in pairs or on their own for part of the activity. Participants are invited to make use of the images provided or to create their own image. This might be a painting or collage that represents the processes they would want to see as core to the way the vision work is taken forward. They can choose to work on their own, in pairs or in small groups. (15–30 mins)

Open gallery viewing and sharing of paintings and collages and the creator's intended message. (15 mins)

Facilitator notes key phrases, metaphors and processes that are talked about during the viewing process. These can be themed and discussed by the group.

A facilitated group discussion about practice development processes. (20–30 mins)

Establish individual and group learning points and relationship to practice development.

Summary and agreed actions. (5 mins)

A key question that can be used in this workshop or group session is 'What matters to you about the way you work with others to realise the shared vision?' The themes, ground-rules or group contract need to feature in any practice development strategy or action plans, and can be used by the practice development coordinating group in future meetings and workshops.

Sheet 3.12: What do we do next?

Suggestions for those who are leading/coordinating the practice developments

Earlier we explained that a shared vision statement sets out the hopes or aspirations for the practice development. It gives us our direction of travel and points us all in the same direction. The temptation is to go dashing off to begin the action. But before you set off, you all need to plan carefully. You need to know where you are starting from because that will help you to see the areas in the workplace and in yourselves that you need to focus on in the development.

The first thing you need to do is to develop a plan to evaluate your starting point, then you can develop an integrated action and evaluation plan. This is an action plan for how you are going to get there. This is integrated with an evaluation plan that helps you to know when you get there and also how you are progressing through the different stages of the practice development journey. And it is the shared vision statement that gives you the focus for all this planning. In Chapter 4, as preparation for evaluating your starting point, we introduce ideas relating to measuring and evaluation and setting up a practice development group to coordinate the evaluation and subsequent practice development plan. In Chapter 5, we focus on getting the commitment of the people who you will need to work with as you develop and carry out the plans. We present a variety of evaluation methods that can be used to get a clear picture of where you are starting from (and which you can repeat as you journey towards your vision to establish how you are doing).

In summary, when you are really clear about the care your service or care home currently gives (through your evaluation of your starting point) and also clear about what you could be doing and you are not in terms of being person-centred, then you can begin to plan what to do. In Chapter 6, we offer resources to help that action planning.

In the meantime you can start talking about the vision every day. You can do this by:

- talking with people who come into or have contact with the service or who live in the care home and visitors to the home about the new vision and the practice development journey the care setting is preparing to take;
- asking yourselves at handover or report whether the way you gave or received handover/report was person-centred;
- talking together about whether you are seeing any small changes or increase in awareness yet in yourself or others in relation to the vision;
- sharing what people who work in your team or who work and live in your home are saying about the vision;
- evaluating on the spot whether what you and your colleague have just done or said matches the values in the vision;
- regularly referring to the vision when you are making plans together for the next day;
- having a thought or message of the week connected to the shared vision.

Useful websites and resources

These are also available on: www.wiley.com/go/practicedevelopment/workbook

'*To Lead, Create a Shared Vision*' *by* James M. Kouzes *and* Barry Z. Posner: *a short article in the* Harvard Business *Review* (http://hbr.org/2009/01/to-lead-create-a-shared-vision/ar/1).

A series of resources showing how the Chief Nurse for England has been promoting a vision for a model of compassionate care (www.commissioningboard.nhs.uk/tag/nursing-vision/).

The Nursing and Midwifery Council's strategic vision (www.nmc-uk.org/About-us/Our-strategic-vision).

'Vision and Values' and the subsequent report '2020 Vision' from The Queen's Nursing Institute looks back at the heritage of the past 150 years of district nursing and offers insights and predictions about the future of district nursing over the next decade to 2020 (www.qni.org.uk/for_nurses/patient_care/2020_vision).

Chapter 4 Introduction to Measuring Progress and Evaluation

Contents

Introduction: Why measuring and evaluating is important

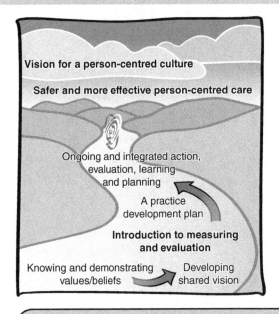

Fig. 4.1 The next step on the practice development journey: Introduction to measuring progress and evaluation.

Chapter 4 starts with information and guidance for those in the care setting coordinating or leading the **practice development**. They can use the information and materials here in their discussions and activities and to explain to the team and patients/residents what evaluation is and how everyone can be involved. The chapter also has a number of learning activities that are specific for direct **care giving team members and housekeeping staff and leaders** in formal roles such as service / ward / care home managers. Some learning tools for **everyone** are also included. Advice for those who are setting up and sustaining a practice development coordinating group is offered. Activities that will be useful to **those leading the evaluation** are also presented.

Practice Development Workbook for Nursing, Health and Social Care Teams, First Edition. Jan Dewing, Brendan McCormack, and Angie Titchen.
© 2014 John Wiley & Sons, Ltd. Published 2014 by John Wiley & Sons, Ltd.
Companion website: www.wiley.com/go/practicedevelopment/workbook

At the end of Chapter 3, we stress the importance of a careful beginning to the practice development journey and the need not to rush into action. This is especially difficult if the visioning activities have made you eager to bring in changes fast. But if you spend time measuring and evaluating where you are starting from, then you will be able to identify areas of strengths and potential to build on and areas of weakness that you need to address. Measuring and evaluating where you and your team stand now will save you a lot of time later because your action will be more focused and more effective. You will make fewer mistakes and take fewer blind alleys. And you will have evidence to show what you are achieving and to convince those who might be sceptical.

Now whilst this careful, measured beginning might sound rather boring, it is far from that. What happens is we discover more things about ourselves, each other and the care setting than we ever knew. For example, we find out that what we thought patients/residents wanted or experienced is sometimes completely different and that patients/residents may see things in entirely different ways to the team! Becoming aware of this difference begins to change us and the care we give. And funnily enough, the *way* we find things out, in addition to *what* we find out, also begins to work a change within us and the ways we work with others. This is because it gives us more insight into ourselves, others and our interactions. All of these processes are part of learning to be more person-centred. So within practice development, measuring and evaluating things are also means of developing ourselves, our leadership and our team-working; to make the ways we work together with co-workers and patients/residents more person-centred. And another thing, the kind of evaluation that we will be introducing you to in this chapter is very different from the kind of measuring and evaluation that often goes on in care settings and care homes. First of all, it is a continuous process, not just at the beginning and end of a project, but all the way through. It is also different because you, team members and patients/residents, if they wish, will be doing it together yourselves and you will be deciding – together – what to do with the new understandings. No one is going to do the measuring and evaluating for you and then tell you what to do. The resources in Chapter 5 will help you learn how to do it.

Finally, some words about audit and evaluation and the differences between them that can help you to answer any questions that others in the care setting might put to you. Audit and evaluation are usually associated with quality assurance, quality improvement and service development. There the focus tends to be on organisational systems and processes. In practice development, evaluation is also concerned with patterns of decision-making, relationships between people, conflict, power use and learning. The key component of audit is that performance is reviewed (or audited) against pre-existing standards to ensure that what should be done is being done, and if not, it provides a framework to enable improvements to be made. In audit and quality assurance work there is often a manager or external auditor who comes in and collects or extracts information from the care setting and takes it away. It may be months before a report comes back, by which time the team might not be able to relate to the original data collection or the report is presented in such a way that it doesn't have meaning for the local team. So what happens in audit is that something is measured against specific evidence-based or value-based standards and that measurement is then positioned along a continuum of met, partially met or not met.

Evaluation, on the other hand, is linked with specific evaluation questions about what is working, for whom and how and in what circumstances. It has to do with the making of a value judgement against explicit criteria derived from the evaluation questions based on where someone or something is along a continuum. This value judgement enables the care setting/home to make decisions about what needs to be prioritised and developed. So whilst both audit and evaluation are concerned with measuring someone or something against criteria from a set of standards and/or research evidence, evaluation is also a systematic determination of merit, worth and significance of the evaluation findings. In other words, whilst both audit and evaluation have a beneficial role to play in developing the working practices of staff, evaluation takes audit a step further.

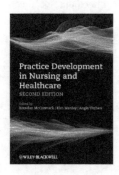

In practice development evaluation, it is vital, as part of active workplace learning and in order to build up the skills set and sustainability in the care setting, that the measuring and evaluation is done by the team members or their peers and in care homes by staff and the people who live there (if they wish) themselves rather than by an external auditor or evaluator. So it will be the staff and patients/residents who determine the significance of audits carried out by others (that are available to you) – any measurements of say, sickness rate, recruitment and retention that are already collected by the organisation – and the new evidence you collect. For the new evidence, you might decide to use the person-centred practice framework (see Chapter 1) or the effective workplace culture concept analysis (see Chapter 5) as the criteria against which you make your judgements. These will be judgements that you make as you travel towards creating person-centred systems, culture and processes that will support person-centred care. For a full account of how evaluation works in practice development, you might like to read two chapters of McCormack et al. (2013). In chapter 9 Sally Hardy, Val Wilson and Tanya McCance set out various perspectives on evaluation and different approaches and methods that can be used. Then in chapter 10 Brendan McCormack, Tanya McCance and Jill Maben describe ways of evaluating outcomes in the development of person-centred practice. These chapters will help with your understanding of the field of evaluation in practice development overall.

If all this sounds daunting, remember, you are not alone on this journey and it is not all done at once. Everyone will be learning and working together in one way or another, over time, in ways that support the evolution of person-centredness in the care setting. Additionally, by networking you will learn from others.

Before you get to the point of familiarising yourself with measuring and evaluation tools and methods, we recommend that the following phases have taken place in your care setting:

1. working out the shared values and beliefs and vision for the stakeholders and service;
2. converting the key purposes into vision statements.

See Chapters 2 and 3 for ideas, guidance, learning activities and tools.

Resources in this chapter

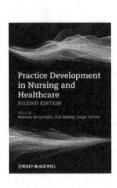

- **Short workshops and/or reflective activities** for starting to think about measuring and evaluation with stakeholders. Stakeholders are people who have an interest or 'stake' in the development or who are 'touched' by or who come into contact with it.
    - **Current methods within your organisation** – this 30 minute workshop helps team members to think about what methods are currently used in the care setting or home to measure and evaluate the service offered. The purpose is to bring to the surface and share questions that people have about measuring and evaluation.
    - **Metrics** – we explain what this buzzword means and give you examples of how metrics might be useful to you as you describe and evaluate your starting point on the practice development journey.
    - **Practice development principles** – we present the key principles that will guide you as you plan and carry out your evaluation and give you some examples of these principles in action, including how to be collaborative, inclusive and participative (CIP principles).
- **Learning activities** – a selection of activities for different team members and care staff groups that can be done by the individual, with a learning buddy and/or with a small group. These simple activities will help prepare you for looking at the measuring and evaluation methods in Chapter 5.
- **Reflection tools** (available on the companion website) – a set of more challenging tools to help you learn how to evaluate your own practice, learn from it and develop plans for learning and improving.
- **An activity for identifying key stakeholders** in the service or care home.
- **A template for a communication plan** – for encouraging stakeholders' commitment.
- **Setting up and sustaining a practice development coordinating group** – in Chapter 3, guidance for a visioning activity group was given. At this stage of the practice development journey, that group may have become, or becomes part of, a coordinating group with a remit for the whole practice development journey in the setting or home. Points to consider when setting up the group, negotiating roles and running it efficiently are offered. In deciding whether to have such a group or not, you might like to read Chapter 5 of McCormack et al. (2013). In this chapter, Brendan McCormack and Jan Dewing show how a practice development coordinating group worked with every part of a national programme of work in Ireland.
- **Working with stakeholders**
    - **Getting at stakeholders' views** – this is a simple resource setting out a method that enables stakeholders' views in the form of their *claims, concerns and issues* about the development to be identified and recorded, even when the stakeholders are in different places.
    - **An example of claims, concerns and issues** – two worked up examples are given: the first about a stroke care service and the second about implementing person-centred dementia care and to show how this tool can be used to develop evaluation questions that will guide the evaluation. However, just like the values and beliefs template in Chapter 2, this template can focus on anything to do with work and the way you and team members work, such as:
        - evaluation of your role;
        - evaluation of part of a service or a whole service offered;
        - evaluation of a group's or meeting's effectiveness;
        - ongoing exploration of the effectiveness of a project or piece of work.
    - **Guidance on facilitating claims, concerns and issues**

In Chapter 9, there are some Frequently Asked Questions that might be relevant *when you are getting started on measuring and evaluating.*

Workshop guidance: Current evaluation methods within your organisation

Guide for a new facilitator

The purpose of this short workshop is to help stakeholders (team members, care home team, patients, residents, families, volunteers and clinical or team leaders) to identify and pool together what each person already knows, their ideas and experiences. It will also help people to think about what they already know and have experienced about measuring quality and evaluation in the service or care home and to identify the questions they have about measuring and evaluation as they set out on the practice development journey together.

You will need:

- 30–45 minutes;
- a facilitator (from within the team);
- a space with a circle of chairs;
- a flipchart and pens;
- sticky notes.

Key activities

Preparation – write up the following questions on a piece of flipchart paper:

- What is the focus of the measurement or evaluation?
- How does the focus relate to the vision?
- What evidence or data are collected?
- Why would this evidence or data be collected?
- Who collected the evidence or data?
- How was the evidence/data collected?
- What did the measuring/evaluation tell you?
- How were the team, patients/residents and families/carers involved?

Introduce the purpose of the workshop and explain that this will be a quiet activity for participants to think about what they already know about measurement and evaluation in the care setting or care home. You may need to use the terms 'audit' and/or 'metrics' (see next resource) at this point to help create links. (5 mins).

Then invite participants to choose a current initiative (a policy/service development or quality improvement work of any sort) that is affecting them at the moment. Ask them to identify the main ways in which it is being evaluated and who does the evaluation. Let participants know that you will guide them through this by reading out the questions on the flipchart one by one, leaving a one minute space in between questions for them to think about the answer and to make notes if they wish.

Read out the questions with the one minute spaces. (10 mins)

Then ask participants to identify for themselves what they know about the topic and key question(s) they have about measuring and evaluation as they begin their practice development work. Ask them to write these questions on sticky notes to enable each person to write their own question(s). Invite each person to stick their notes on the flipchart and then view all the questions that have been put forward (5 mins). It can be reassuring to let people know that spelling errors are OK. Occasionally there may be someone who needs support due to language or literacy issues.

Invite participants to reflect on the questions together and share any ideas they have in response to them.

If you have 45 minutes for this workshop then also help them to establish which questions are the most important for them to address. Suggest that they might like to think about how they could find out what they need to know and make some action points (see the following table).

Possible actions that come up during the workshop

Action points (What specifically will you do?)	Agreed completion date	New skills/knowledge needed? (Detail how these will be acquired)

Keep a record of the participants' questions (and action points if you have had time to do them). After gaining workshop participants' permission, give them (along with the date of the workshop and who facilitated it) to the practice development group who is coordinating the evaluation (see Chapter 5). The questions (and action points) are likely to be useful in helping the group determine how stakeholders in the service or care home will need to be prepared for gathering and analysing evaluation evidence.

If there are other people in the service or care home who work in what is referred to as in-reaching or out-reaching, who wanted to attend the workshop but couldn't, you could give them this instruction sheet and invite them to work through it by themselves or by reflecting with their learning buddy. You could also invite them to give you their questions to add to those already gathered in the workshop.

As a follow-up to this workshop, consider organising the small group discussion on measuring and metrics that follows now. The guidance for doing this can be found at www.wiley.com/go/practicedevelopment/workbook

Trigger for group discussion: What are 'metrics' and how do we measure person-centred care?

Guide for a new facilitator to facilitate a discussion in the practice development coordinating group

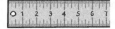

You might have come across the buzz word *metrics* that is around at the moment. This is a term used in relation to the *measurement* of certain core aspects of quality in health and social care. A *metric* means any set or collection of information or evidence, either quantitative or qualitative that is derived from a standard. So, in a care home, a metric could be a set of evidence about, say, residents' well-being, the social activities they engage in, the number of falls residents have had in the past year, or data about residents who experience difficulties with eating and associated weight control. In health care, metrics often include measures of infection, pressure sores, falls, clinical incidents and length of stay. The term *metrics* then refers to more than one set of information or evidence. When the sets are put together in one tool they are often referred to as a 'dashboard'.

Perhaps you have already identified metrics in your service or care home that have been collected to measure the quality of care? What are they?

An *indicator* (another term that is frequently used) is a particular sort of metric that indicates issues or areas that may be worth investigating and might show that other related areas of care are not as good as they should be. For example, if patient satisfaction or residents' well-being scores had dropped or the number of falls or the number of patients /residents being prescribed neuroleptic medications was very much higher than in previous years, then the managers would probably want to examine why – or you would be asked to help with an examination.

We have chosen as examples relatively simple things that are relatively easy to record and count. However, *measuring* whether care is person-centred or not, and whether the climate or culture in the care setting or care home is supporting that kind of care or not, is not so easy. This is because there are so many different things to measure and influencing factors to take into account. Fortunately for us, some simple tools have been developed and we will be offering some of those to you in Chapter 5.

The discussion could focus on what metrics and indicators are available in your care setting or care home and which ones might be the most useful for evaluating the starting point towards your shared vision.

You may need to identify a few new metrics. Your suggested new measures might be different from the ones collected up to this point.

OR

Invite the coordinating group members to relook at the vision statement (if this has already been done) and see what metrics you can develop from this.

Note: any new metrics must be back-tracked and linked to a standard.

Trigger for group discussion: Practice development principles for measuring and evaluation

Guide for a new facilitator to facilitate a discussion in the practice development coordinating group

In the introduction to this resource, we gave a definition and framework for practice development (see Chapter 1). So building on them, we see the principles of practice development work in general as follows.
Practice development is:

- based on working towards a shared common vision;
- a continuous process of improvement and innovation towards person-centred care and transformation of the workplace culture and organisation of care;
- brought about by teams developing their knowledge and skills through reflection and work-based learning;
- helped by teams being committed to systematic, rigorous and continuous processes of change that help us get round the obstacles that get in the way of us achieving our shared vision;
- person-centred and reflects the perspectives of the people who receive care or live there and families and carers.

In relation to measuring and evaluation, these general principles translate as:

- An evaluation plan is guided by the shared vision of all the stakeholders and is developed by them (CIP: collaboration, inclusion and participation).
- Teams learn how to work together in person-centred ways. They learn how to help stakeholders to collaborate, participate and be included in the planning and its implementation.
- Efforts towards increasing the effectiveness and person-centredness of care and transforming the workplace culture and way care is organised are regularly and systematically measured and evaluated by stakeholders.
- The methods used to gather data are person-centred and help to advance the development as well as provide metrics and indicators to evaluate it.
- Stakeholders evaluate their own participation in the process, and reflect on and learn from the obstacles inside themselves that may be slowing down or preventing the development of person-centred care.

In your small group, you could discuss these principles and relate them to your own service or care home. Another activity could be discussion about the following example of metrics.

Example of possible metrics

Mulberry Unit is a 20 bedded day surgery unit. The team have recently started exploring their own practice and have just completed their vision statement. They are now looking at how their care and practice is evaluated, by whom and how useful these measures are. The group members went on a fact-finding mission and discovered that the following metrics were collected:

- pressure sores/skin integrity;
- wrist bands in place;
- falls;
- infection levels;
- complaints;
- serious incidents reported correctly.

Following discussion the group members identified the top three measures they wanted to explore:

- pain management
- patient experience
- discharge process (to include information sharing)

They shared their ideas via a colourful poster with the rest of the team to seek their support to take the work forward.

Meadow Lodge is a care home with 35 people living there, most of whom have dementia. A small group from the team facilitated by a Registered Mental Health Nurse (RMN) discovered what metrics currently exist in their home and how these are reported. The group feels that a few new metrics could be introduced; for example, agitation levels, pain management and end-of-life care.

The group came to this view after relooking at their new vision statement in which they state:

> The purpose of our care at Meadow Lodge is to enable people living here to feel well, express themselves and their choices and be free of pain and discomfort especially at the end of their lives.

Enderby ward is an acute medial admissions ward with 32 beds. Older people form the main service users and many people (45% at least) have a diagnosis of dementia or delirium. A small group within the nursing and therapy team and the housekeeping team were exploring their values and beliefs about the care of people with dementia and delirium. They watched a TV programme extract in which Jo Brand discusses a scheme to help tackle poor dementia care in hospitals (a leaflet called 'This is me') so the patient's details are known to hospital staff (www.youtube.com/watch?v=WDjO52OUXGM).

After discussion, the team members decided that as well as introducing the 'This Is ME' document, they needed a new metric to find out whether antipsychotic medication was used unnecessarily in the ward.

They invited a Dementia Care Champion from a neighbouring ward and a community RMN to come and work with them in gathering the baseline or current evidence and used it eventually to use more creative approaches for minimising the use of these drugs. The ward pharmacist was asked to help with collecting the evidence from prescriptions.

Learning activity for teams: Evaluating care plans

This learning activity is for all team members

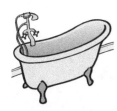

The purpose of this activity is to show you how evaluation can be carried out in ways that bring about opportunities for learning and development at the same time. The activity can be done alone, with a learning buddy or with a small group of team members.

You will need:

- about 30 minutes if you are doing it alone or with a buddy and an extra 30 minutes (can be on a different day) if you are doing it with a small group;
- access to the care plans of the people you personally look after;
- this instruction sheet;
- a quiet space in which to reflect.

Key activities
Negotiate with your fellow workers to have time to look at the records of five people who you work with or have worked with recently.

Examine the care records and fill in the following form (tick Yes or No for each person). When you have answered the questions add up the number of Yes/No answers for each person.

Please see the form on the next page – we have put it on a page on its own in case you want to copy it. There is also plenty of space on the page for you to write examples of what you find to support your Yes or No selection.

For each question indicate **Yes** or **No** in the boxes in appropriate column and row:

Question	Person 1 Yes/No	Person 2 Yes/No	Person 3 Yes/No	Person 4 Yes/No	Person 5 Yes/No
Does the assessment/care plan indicate:					
1. what matters to the person?					
2. the person's preferences about personal care?					
3. whether a shower or bath is preferred?					
4. the person's particular food preferences ?					
Total number of Yes/No responses					

My notes:

If you are on your own or with your learning buddy or clinical supervisor, reflect on:

- what your results mean in relation to your own care of that person (e.g. if you have more No than Yes responses, think about why that might be);
- how you feel about the results;
- what sense you make of them;
- whether you have ever looked at the assessments before;
- if you have, whether you have paid attention to the person's stated preferences in the daily care you provide;
- how you take into account who the person is as you give personal care;
- whether you need to take some action as a result of this measurement and evaluation and develop action points.

If you are doing this activity with a small group, take turns to share or present your results and your action points. See if you can learn from each other's ideas and plans.

Remember, this is a learning activity and no blame should be attributed to anyone having No responses. The idea is to support each other, to discuss the meaning of the findings for each of you and also for the service or home overall and to see if some collective action could be taken to improve care.

Example 1

Margaret works as a Support Worker (Level 3) in her team. From working through this activity Margaret realises she does not look at the initial nursing assessments. She also noted that the care plans are kept in a different place than the assessment information. Neither is kept with the patients. She tends to rely on the handover sheet she is given at the start of her shift. Her action point is to look through assessments and to start asking other team members about where the care plans could better be kept.

Example 2

Rosie works in a care home as a care assistant. From working through this activity she realises that she does not look at the care plans and relies on what other staff in the home tell her. Her action point is to look through care plans on a monthly basis with support from one of the Registered Nurses (RN).

Note: We are not suggesting that this is all you need to do to evaluate care plans – this is meant as a short learning activity that incorporates a small practical aspect of measurement.

You could also select other topics for this activity, such as sleep, pain, special occasions and end-of-life care including after death care.

Learning activity for teams: Evaluating your respect for dignity, privacy and the control people have in your service

This learning activity is for all team members

Like the previous activity, the purpose of this activity is to show you how evaluation can be carried out in ways that bring about opportunities for learning and development at the same time. The activity can be done alone, with your learning buddy or with a small group of health-care assistants or carers.

You will need:

- 15 minutes;
- this instruction sheet;
- a notebook or piece of paper and pen;
- a quiet space in which to reflect.

Key activities

Please see the questionnaire on the next page – we have put it on a page on its own in case you want to copy it.

Ask yourself the questions below. Tick one response for each question and then count up the number of ticks in each column.

Offering personal care	Yes	No	Sometimes
If they are in a single room, do I knock on the person's door and wait for a response before I enter?			
Do I plan my work to fit in with the person's preferences for the time they wish to get up in the morning?			
If there are visitors in the ward/rooms, do I rearrange my plans so as not to disturb them?			
Do I negotiate with people what time they would like their care?			
If I am unable to make the time we negotiated, do I return to the person to make other arrangements?			
Do I ensure dignity and privacy when giving personal care?			
Do I shut the toilet door when it is in use?			
Do I ask people where they would like their personal effects or flowers placed, if I have had to move them in the course of the care?			
Do I ask permission to enter shared areas/bays?			
Do I encourage people to be as independent as possible?			
Do I encourage people to contribute to making decisions for themselves if they want to, in the way they want to?			
Do I know how people with expressive communication or cognitive impairment (such as advanced dementia) communicate their choices and preferences?			
Total number of Yes/No/Sometimes responses			

If you are on your own or with your learning buddy, reflect on:

- what your results mean in relation to the care you offer patients/residents (e.g. if you have more No than Yes responses, think about why that might be);
- how you feel about the results;
- what sense you make of them;
- whether you need to take some action as a result of this measurement and evaluation;
- what support you might need to be able to take the action(s).

If you are doing this activity with a small group, take turns to present your results and your action points. See if you can learn from each other's ideas and points.

Remember, this is a learning activity and no blame should be attributed to anyone for having No responses. The idea is to support each other, to discuss the meaning of the findings for each of you and also for the service or home overall, and to see whether some collective action could be taken to improve care.

Examples

Marie has been asked to notice how privacy and dignity are maintained by the ward team. This was an action for everyone at the recent practice development group. She thought it was not an issue on her ward. However, she now is noticing several aspects that could be improved on. On one morning this week, Marie saw nurses and therapists going into rooms and behind screens without knocking or announcing who they were. She twice saw team members going into toilets without asking the patient's permission. She was also aware that a few doctors arrived to see patients in the middle of their lunch. Marie will be sharing her observations, along with the good aspects she also noticed, with the group at their next session.

Saurav works as a housekeeper at Maytree House. He always tries to ask people if he can go in to clean their rooms. He has a plan of what each person particularly likes done. Sometimes he asks people to check whether they are satisfied with the cleaning. He feels that they should have more say in how their rooms and possessions are looked after. The manager has discovered this from a few of the residents and would like Saurav to talk to the team about this as a learning activity.

Learning activity for teams: Cats, skirts, handbags and lipstick

This learning activity is for all care home team members

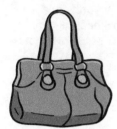

Developed by a participant (Deirdre Ryan, St Mary's Care Centre, Mullingar, Republic of Ireland) in the practice development programme, *The Implementation of a Model of Person-Centred Practice in Older Person Settings* (McCormack et al. 2010), the *cats, skirts, handbags and lipstick activity* has helped care staff to develop much more person-centred care plans for residents that now include the things that matter to residents. Doing the activity helped participants to recognise that there were things they did not know about the people living there and that they probably had not really considered. They found that many of the things that people would like were quite small and achievable, like a request to 'give me my make-up bag and handbag in the morning and leave me to put it on myself' to 'I have never worn trousers in my life, please don't try to make me wear them now'.

You may find that some people are quite surprised that they haven't been asked before:

> They should have been asked when admitted 'what is' and 'what was important' to them, not after a few months or years later about what could make life better for you here (Older person)
>
> (McCormack et al., 2010)

Would you like to try this simple learning and evaluation activity?
You will need:

- 15–20 minutes;
- a notebook and pen;
- a private, quiet and comfortable place to sit with a resident and have a structured conversation.

Key activities In advance of the conversation with the older person and to get their permission, explain to them that, as part of the practice development in the care home, all staff are trying to centre their care on the needs of the people living there. You could say that you would therefore like to hear what is important to them and ask them whether they would be willing to tell you, so that it can be included in their care plan. Tell them that you will structure the conversation around four things that are important to them on a daily basis. Reassure them that if they don't want to talk with you, you will respect that and no one will hold it against them in any way.

When you meet for the conversation, explain again what you are doing and check that they are still OK with it.

Then ask them to identify the four key things that on a daily basis they need/like/want in order to feel 'good'. These things can be as simple as salt on my food, more sugar in my tea, be able to go outside, wear shoes with heels and not slippers and so on.

After you have finished the conversation and thanked them, take a few minutes alone to reflect on what the resident has said and ask yourself whether you knew these things already and if you didn't, ask yourself why. Think for a moment about how you could incorporate these four things into your care for that person.

On another occasion, if other carers are doing this activity, arrange to meet together to share the four things that have arisen. There is likely to be a huge range of things. Discuss how you can all get to know what each person likes and how the team can make sure that the care it gives includes what makes the person feel good.

Finding ways to know the individual preferences of persons we are providing care to is really important in being person-centred. Visit **www.wiley.com/go/practicedevelopment/workbook** for an example of a process called 'At a Glance' associated with this chapter. This process enables care workers to make explicit the person's individual preferences in their care plan.

Learning activity for staff who serve food & drink: Evaluating the service you offer

This activity is designed for members of the team including volunteers and anyone else who serve meals and refreshments. Depending on how your care setting or home operates this might be support staff or care workers.

The purpose of the activity is to show you how evaluation can be carried out in ways that bring about opportunities for learning and improvement at the same time. The activity can be done on your own, with your learning buddy or with a small group of catering or housekeeping staff.

You will need:

- 15 minutes;
- this instruction sheet;
- a notebook or piece of paper and pen;
- a quiet space to think in.

Please see the questionnaire on the next page – we have put it on a page on its own in case you want to copy it.

If you serve people their meals and drinks, ask yourself the questions below. Tick a Yes/No response for each question and then count up the number of ticks in each column.

Serving meals and drinks	Yes	No	Sometimes
Do we know what kind of food and drink each person likes?			
Do we know what kind of food and drink each person dislikes?			
Do we ensure that each person has a choice in what they eat or drink?			
Do we know the amount of food each person likes to have?			
Do we make sure each person can reach their food and drink?			
Do we make use of red trays* for food and red lids* for water jugs?			
If someone has not touched their food, do I just take it away without informing the appropriate person?			
Do we provide a positive environment and atmosphere for each person to have meals in?			
Do we regularly ask each person for feedback on their meals?			
Do we evaluate patients/residents' satisfaction with the menu?			
Total number of Yes/No/Sometimes responses			

* see this link for further information: www.rcn.org.uk/development/practice/cpd_online_learning/supporting _peoples_nutritional_needs/supporting_and_assisting_people

My notes:

Now reflect on:

- what your results mean in relation to your own care of that person (e.g. if you have more 'No' than 'Yes' responses, think about why that might be);
- how you feel about the results;
- what sense you make of them;
- whether you need to take some action as a result of this measurement and evaluation and develop some action points.

If you are doing this activity with your buddy or a small group, take turns to present your results and your action points. See if you can learn from each other's ideas and points.

Remember, this is a learning activity and no blame should be attributed to anyone for having 'no' responses. The idea is to support each other, to discuss the meaning of the findings for each of you and also for the service or home overall and to see whether some collective action could be taken to improve this service.

Example 1

Elsie works in the kitchen and also serves food at mealtimes in the dining room. She feels 'her' people are well cared for. Her buddy has helped her to see that the atmosphere in the dining room can be rushed and noisy. The team like to have the radio on – Elsie had never considered what impact this might have on people with sensory impairments or cognitive impairments. Elsie has agreed to observe the effects and whether it effects the residents' enjoyment of their meals.

Example 2

As part of a Trust-wide peer audit of red trays and red lids, ward housekeeping staff were asked about use of the trays and lids in their wards. On Tamar ward, Shelia told the nurse auditing that they didn't need these on their ward because the care at mealtimes was good. Shelia intended to show that the nursing team did a good job. However, this isn't how her response was interpreted. When the audit results were fed back it was suggested to the ward manager on Tamar ward that she focused on raising awareness about the purpose of red trays and red lids amongst her whole team.

Learning activity for housekeepers: Evaluating the cleaning, housekeeping or repair service you offer

> This activity is designed for housekeepers

The purpose is to show you how evaluation can be carried out in ways that bring about opportunities for learning and improvement at the same time. The activity can be done alone, with a learning buddy or with a small group of staff.
    You will need:

- 15 minutes;
- this instruction sheet;
- a notebook or piece of paper and pen;
- a quiet space to think in.

Key activities   If you serve people by cleaning or offering housekeeping or repair services, ask yourself the questions below. Tick one response for each question and then count up the number of ticks in each column.
    Please see the next page – we have put the questionnaire on its own page in case you want to copy it.

Cleaning & housekeeping duties	Yes	No	Sometimes
Do I ask the person whether I can clean around their bed area / Do I knock on the person's door and wait for a response before I enter?			
Do I plan my work around the nursing, therapy or personal care the person is having?			
If there are visitors in the bed area or rooms, do I rearrange my plans so as not to disturb them?			
If it is unavoidable that I have to carry out my duties in the person's own bed area/room when they are in it, do I negotiate where they might go whilst the work is carried out and help, or arrange help for, them to get there?			
If it is unavoidable that I have to carry out my duties in the person's own bed area or room when they are in it and they are not well enough to go elsewhere, do I respect their privacy?			
Do I include people in what I'm doing by talking with them as I work?			
Do I ask people whether they are satisfied with the work I do?			
Total number of Yes/No/Sometimes responses			

My notes: What I saw or questions I have

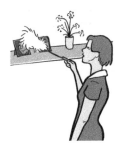

If you are on your own or with a learning buddy, reflect on:

- what your results mean in relation to the service you offer patients/residents (e.g. if you have more No than Yes responses, think about why that might be);
- how you feel about the results;
- what sense you make of them;
- whether you need to take some action as a result of this measurement and evaluation and develop some action points.

If you are doing this activity with a small group, take turns to present your results and your action points. See whether you can learn from each other's ideas and points.

Remember, this is a learning activity and no blame should be attributed to anyone for having No responses. The idea is to support each other, to discuss the meaning of the findings for each of you and also for the service or home overall and to see whether some collective action could be taken to improve services.

Example 1

Marja works as a member of the housekeeping team in a large hospital. She tends to 'fill in' for others, so she is asked to work in many different areas. She enjoys working in the Special Care Baby Unit because she is asked by the Matron to ask the parents and family members to see whether it's convenient for them that she does her work and to see whether they are satisfied with the standard of cleanliness. At first, Marja found this odd as she is not asked to do this anywhere else. After the Matron explained the reason why this is done, Marja appreciated it was a good idea that parents felt confident about the level of privacy for their baby, themselves and the level of cleanliness. She now tries to do this on other wards and it often leads to a nice conversation with patients or families.

Example 2

Martin does repair jobs for a number of homes in the company. In one of the homes one of the men is always pleased to see him and wants to help with jobs and repairs. Although the man (Ted) is pleasant, Martin has always seen Ted as an inconvenience that slows him down due to his cognitive impairment. Martin has learned that team members in the home think Ted should be encouraged to feel useful and valued about the home. The RN suggested to Martin that Ted could be asked to paint as he likes this work. Martin has agreed to help Ted do this on his next visit. The staff will set up a 'pot of paint' (water with food colouring added) and a brush and find something that needs painting.

They all agree to see what effect this has on Ted.

Learning activity for team or home managers and those with an interest in learning and practice development: Evaluating the learning support systems for care teams

This activity is designed for unit/ward/home managers, team leaders or anyone who has responsibility or an interest in learning and practice development within the care setting or care home

The purpose is to show you how evaluation can be carried out in ways that bring about opportunities for learning and improvement at the same time.

You will need:

- 15 minutes;
- this instruction sheet;
- a notebook or piece of paper and pen;
- a quiet space to think in.

Key activities

These questions will help you to think about whether there are systems in place to support work-based learning for teams and if so, whether you are supporting their use. Tick one response for each question and then count up the number of ticks in each column.

Please see the questionnaire on the next page.

Work-based learning	Yes	No	Sometimes
Are there policies for one-to-one learning, like clinical or professional supervision, mentoring or learning buddies?			
Are these formal systems for one-to-one learning in place and being used?			
Are there policies for regular, formal training sessions offered for groups?			
Do I organise or offer training sessions for the team?			
Do we have a range of learning resources available on site?			
Do I encourage informal opportunities for work-based learning, e.g. during the shift handover or ensuring that a new or less experienced member of the team works alongside a more experienced member in the overlap between the early and late shift with the intention of learning?			
Do I encourage informal networking with people working in other similar services or homes to ours?			
Do I have regular opportunities to learn and develop my management and leadership skills?			
Total number of Yes/No/Sometimes responses			

My notes: Comments and questions I have

If you are working on your own, reflect on:

- what your results mean in relation to your management/work-based learning responsibilities;
- how you feel about the results;
- what sense you make of them;
- whether you need to take some action as a result of this measurement and evaluation and develop some action points.

If you are doing this activity with a small group, take turns to present your results and your action points. See whether you can learn from each other's ideas and points.

Remember, this is a learning activity and no blame should be attributed to anyone for having No responses. The idea is to support each other, to discuss the meaning of the findings for each of you and also for the home overall and to see whether some collective action could be taken to improve work-based learning in the care setting.

Guide: Reflection tools

> This guide is for all team members

On several occasions in this resource, we have invited you to reflect on something, for example your values and beliefs and in the measuring and evaluating activities above. Reflection gives you the opportunity to evaluate yourself. That is why we have included the three reflection tools on the companion website. They can help you to reflect more systematically and deeply as you work to become more person-centred through learning and evaluating your own practice. But just a brief word here about reflection to help you get started.

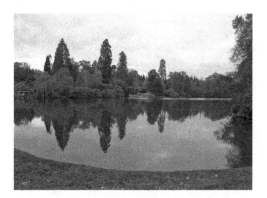

What is reflection?

Reflection is like holding up a mirror to yourself or leaning over a tranquil lake and really looking at yourself and asking yourself questions about what you see. This is sometimes called a dialogue with yourself. You can also have a dialogue with others about what you see and feel as you question and evaluate yourself. Now you may think that reflection is something you do every day. For example, you might mull over your working day as you travel home alone or, as you eat your lunch with a fellow worker, you might talk about an incident or something that happened to you and a resident that morning. But these conversations and stories are likely to be unstructured (they may even be chaotic!) and may not go very deep beneath the surface or they may be unquestioning. So, they may not increase your understanding of yourself as a worker or give you an explanation of the problem that has occurred. Also, they may not help you to evaluate your own part in whatever you are reflecting upon or help you to see what you could do next to improve or resolve an issue or problem. In other words, such reflection might not take you anywhere.

Why should I do it then? Reflection that is structured is more likely to help you to think through an issue, event, situation or problem systematically. Such reflection helps you to question what you have always taken for granted, to think more deeply, to look at things from different angles or 'out of the box'. Sometimes it will challenge, for example, the way you think you are as a worker and the impact you have in your relationships with residents and fellow workers. And structured reflection will help you to devise action points of what you can do next.

How do I do it? Structured reflection can be done on your own or with others. For instance, if you have done any of the learning activities above, you will already have experienced doing structured reflection. First you will have responded alone to the questions posed in the activity (a dialogue with yourself) and then you will have discussed them and maybe some action points with your buddy or the small group (a dialogue with others). It is likely that in the dialogue with others, your understanding developed further and you might have been able to refine your action points or get new ideas of what to do.

What will I get out of it? By increasing your ability to reflect and evaluate yourself more effectively, you will be better able to contribute to the practice development journey to improving the culture of your workplace and ultimately to person-centredness. You will become a more effective worker by reflecting upon and evaluating:

- how you make decisions about your work, for example do I share decision-making with patients/residents?
- the part you play in keeping the culture and context in the service or home the same, or in developing it to make it more person-centred;
- the ways you relate to others, use power, deal with conflict or learn in and from work.

You are likely to become more committed to developing yourself, overcoming obstacles/resistance in yourself and in the context of things that are getting in the way of person-centred practice and improving the care/service you give to residents and families. Potentially, you could develop more satisfying and productive working relationships with colleagues and the satisfaction of contributing to something bigger.

What is in it for people for whom I provide care/services?   If team members develop as above, then patients/residents are likely to feel that their needs, as they see them, are met. Their values will be included in decision-making about their care and environment, they will feel genuinely listened to and they will flourish. Their identity as a person will be maintained and they will live with dignity and respect.

> In a nutshell, structured reflection is vital for the practice development journey. If team members are not reflective and do not evaluate their own actions, then it is unlikely that the vision statements will be achieved. Making the journey to person-centred care is dependent on reflective teams. Practice development is deeply tied to learning in and from work and to evaluating that learning in order to improve, to change, and to flourish. Chapter 8 of this resource is all about making such learning happen in the care home.

Now visit **www.wiley.com/go/practicedevelopment/workbook** where you will find three different reflective tools. These tools were first published in Dewing & Titchen (2007). Completed examples for tools 1 and 2 have been developed as a way of helping you make best use of the tools and develop your reflection skills.

Getting the commitment of stakeholders

This activity is for the practice development coordinating group (if there is one) and/or for those who are interested in being involved in evaluation.

Everyone in the care setting and those associated with it in some way will be 'touched' by the evaluation and action and so are potential stakeholders. Ideally, everyone will be involved over time, but it is likely that people will want to be included and participate in varying degrees and ways and at different times. There will also be people who have a bigger part to play. We call these people key stakeholders. The purpose of this activity is, first, to identify who you think are the key stakeholders that you will have to work with directly in evaluating the starting point on your practice development journey, then to establish those you need to consult or inform. Second, the activity will help you to develop a communication plan to engage with these stakeholders.

You can do this activity in a small, informal group with someone taking the lead to structure the activities.

You will need:

- 20–30 minutes;
- a copy of this sheet of instructions;
- a room in the care home with chairs for people to sit;
- a flipchart and pens.

Key activities

On the flipchart sheet, write a list of the names of everyone the group thinks are key stakeholders. Help them to think widely as there are likely to be individuals or services that might not at first come to mind, but who might influence the development of person-centred care or be affected by it. Such people might turn out to be your biggest support or be the biggest resisters to change. Stick this flipchart sheet on the wall if possible.

- Now draw three circles – one inside the other on a new sheet.
- Identify who in the list are your key stakeholders that you need to work directly with and write their names in the centre circle (see example below).
- In the next circle going out, write the names of those you need to consult.
- And in the next circle, those you need to keep informed and establish communication channels.
- Check that you have included everyone on the list in one of the circles.

The next step is to develop a communication plan with these different kinds of stakeholders and to establish who will be responsible for what. The following template will be helpful here. For example, one of the stakeholders that you will work with *directly* is the patient or the resident committee. If one of the stakeholders that you need to *consult* is very senior in the organisation, then you may need support from the manager to do this with them. And if one of the stakeholders that you need to *inform* is the external supplier of a service, then the person who liaises with that supplier might be the person to ask.

After the activity the template should be filled in and circulated to the group for checking.

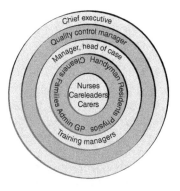

Template for developing a communication plan with stakeholders

Who are our stakeholders?	How best to do this?	Who will communicate?
Those we will work with directly (these people might become members of the practice development coordinating group)		
Those you will consult		
Those you will inform		

Guide: Setting up and sustaining a practice development coordinating group[1]

> This guide is for the people who are interested in setting up a practice development coordinating group. They are likely to be some of the key stakeholders identified in the previous activity. Some people are likely to be team members with professional or vocational qualifications, others are likely to be patients/residents and other team members who are interested in being involved.

Setting up a practice development coordinating group enables more efficiency, effectiveness and success of the practice development journey. In larger organisations it can be seen as part of clinical governance or various quality improvement work or programmes. For example, a service manager or Head of Nursing or Matron may set up this sort of group to help develop consistency in practice development across several wards, departments or community teams. It is likely to be set up after the vision statement has been created and the key stakeholders have been identified. A decision will need to be made about which of the key stakeholders would be best to invite onto the coordinating group. You will need to think about the following when making your decision.

- The purpose of practice development coordinating is to lead, oversee and coordinate the evaluation of where we are starting from in our practice development journey in the services or care home. From there, the purpose is to lead on the practice development plan, which includes integrating actions and their evaluation, learning and replanning.
- Who amongst the key stakeholders that have been identified have embraced the shared vision with enthusiasm?
- Who has the skills, capacity and potential willingness to join the group?
- How can we ensure that group membership reflects the spread of key stakeholders?
- How big a group do we need?
- How often will the group need to meet, where and at what time?
- Who will take the group lead or coordination role?
- How will the work of the group be resourced?

Once the group is established, group members will need to:

- discuss and agree the remit of the group;
- clarify their roles within the group (see Chapter 3) and negotiate these roles with other group members;
- establish ground rules or person-centred ways of working together (see Chapter 2 for a handout).

Group members may also wish to review the questions (and action points) generated by stakeholders at the workshop on *Current evaluation methods within your organisation* (see Chapter 5) to get a sense of where stakeholders are starting from in terms of the practice development journey.

The templates for efficient agenda setting and note-taking, presented in Chapter 3 could be modified for this meeting. Other examples of agendas are provided at **www.wiley.com/go/practicedevelopment/workbook**, showing how progress on actions are monitored and replanned if necessary.

If you are working with a practice development coordinating group, then having processes in place to ensure stakeholder engagement is important. We recognise that the next sections in this resource are based on the assumption that a practice development coordinating group will have been set up in the care setting. If you decide not to do this, you might still like to look through these sections and see whether there are any ideas you can draw on in your work.

---

[1] Whilst we strongly recommend the setting up of such an overview practice development group, we recognise that this may not be possible or seen as desirable in some settings or care homes. The rest of this resource is still relevant for individuals and groups of co-workers (and patients and residents who are working together to improve the experience of care and services). We continue to offer individual and group activities as well as more formal ones.

Claims, Concerns and Issues: An evaluation tool for working with stakeholders
(Guba & Lincoln, 1989)

> This guide is offered for any kind of group wanting to involve stakeholders in their work and evaluations

Used at the outset and all the way through the practice development journey, the Claims, Concerns and Issues (CCIs) evaluation tool helps stakeholders to be included and to collaborate and participate in the practice development in an effective person-centred way. Like the values and beliefs clarification activity in Chapter 2, this activity, when carried out well, is democratic in that it helps everybody's voice to be heard and be taken into account in the discussion.

Claims are positive or favourable statements about the topic being discussed. Concerns are any negative or unfavourable assertions about the topic. Issues are questions that reflect what any 'reasonable person' might ask about the topic, and usually emerge from concerns. The facilitator records the stakeholders' concerns, and then invites them to reconsider their concerns and frame them as questions, thus providing more issues that can be explored in whatever work that follows. **These questions can later be worked up as evaluation questions that will guide the evaluation planning and implementation (see Chapter 5).**

Stakeholders can put forward any statement about claims, concerns or issues they wish. However, once they are all proposed, the statements must be open to constructive discussion by others.

If you want to use CCIs with the different stakeholder groups, it is important that you identify all the possible groups that need to be involved and agree how you will get a balance of representation within each of the groups.

CCIs can be carried out as part of a formal evaluation of practice development, as we are suggesting at this point in the resource, or within various elements of practice development work. For example, CCIs can be used regularly as part of practice development meetings and groups to either set agendas or as one item on an agenda. Individual practice developers and practitioners can also use CCIs as part of the self-assessment of their practice.

A template for stakeholders' views: Claims, Concerns and Issues

CLAIMS: What positive statements would I make about . . . .?

_____

_____

_____

_____

_____

_____

_____

_____

_____

_____

_____

_____

_____

_____

_____

_____

_____

CONCERNS: What are my concerns about . . . .?

_____

_____

_____

_____

_____

_____

_____

_____

_____

_____

_____

_____

_____

_____

_____

_____

_____

ISSUES: What questions do I have about . . . .?

_____

_____

_____

_____

_____

_____

_____

_____

_____

_____

_____

_____

_____

_____

_____

_____

_____

Participants' resources, Practice Development School, London: International Practice Development Collaborative (unpublished work taken from Guba and Lincoln, 1989). A more detailed account of Guba & Lincoln's work on Fourth Generation Evaluation (from which Claims, Concerns and Issues are derived) can be found in Chapter 9 of McCormack et al. (2013).

An example of Claims, Concerns and Issues (1)

My claims about our integrated multi-professional documentation and the way it works are:
   (These are positive statements that one team member has presented)

It looks professional
It's the same in all wards and teams
Everything is in one place
Nothing falls out
It follows the patient journey
It's better than what we used before
All professions contribute to it
It's easier for auditing
It's more organised for investigating complaints

My concerns about our integrated **multi-**professional documentation and the way it works are:
   (These are statements about the less-than-positive feelings you have about it.)

It's too big
Too much paper work
Not enough time to do all the assessments
Doctors don't always use it
Some teams have changed it
Some teams have introduced other paperwork
There's no training for new staff on how to use it

My issues about our integrated **multi-**professional documentation and the way it works are:
   (These are reasonable questions you have wanted to ask, but haven't so far, or you've tried to ask but haven't been heard.)

Why do we have to have so much paperwork?
How can we reduce the amount of documentation we have to do?
How do we get everyone to use the same documents?
How do we know what the quality of documentation is?
What is our governance here?

Note: These are only one person's CCIs. They would need to be combined with other stakeholders' CCIs to enable all stakeholders to see the range of CCIs and to identify where they are shared. The idea is to generate a list of issues or questions from everyone's concerns (so that all the concerns are converted into questions).

An example of Claims, Concerns and Issues (2)

My claims about person-centred dementia care and the way it works are:
(These are positive statements that one team member has presented)

*I've heard people say it respects persons with dementia and makes them
feel valued
I feel I would learn a lot of new skills to provide it
I have read good things about person-centred dementia care on the Alzheimer's Society website
I feel open to the idea and to trying it out for our home*

My concerns about person-centred dementia care and the way it works are:
(These are statements about the less-than-positive feelings you have about it.)

*I don't have any previous experience of person-centred dementia care
I feel anxious about knowing how to do it or what to do
I can't see how I can fit it in, as this kind of care takes a lot of time
I'm worried my skills aren't good enough*

My issues about person-centred dementia care and the way it works are:
(These are reasonable questions you have wanted to ask, but haven't so far, or you've tried to ask but haven't been heard.)

*What if I don't like the person with dementia?
How can we find the time to develop it?
How can I get the skills to do person-centred dementia care?*

Note: These are only one person's CCIs. They would need to be combined with other stakeholders' CCIs to enable all stakeholders to see the range of CCIs and to identify where they are shared. For example, if they are shared:

I don't have any previous experience of person-centred dementia care

becomes

What sort of experiences do we need to have to start giving person-centred dementia care?

I feel anxious about knowing how to do it or what to do

becomes

How can we prepare ourselves to start being person-centred with older people who have dementia?

I can't see how I can fit it in, as this kind of care takes a lot of time

becomes

How do we create and/or negotiate the time needed for person-centred care in our work?

How can I get the skills to do person-centred dementia care?

becomes

How will active learning help us to develop our skills?

Guide: Facilitating Claims, Concerns and Issues (adapted from Dewing & Titchen, 2007)

This guide is for the practice development coordinating group and for other groups that are set up during the practice development journey

At the start of the practice development journey, the purpose of conducting a CCIs activity is to be person-centred by involving stakeholders in the journey so they have their say about it. It is also to gather evidence to help stakeholders to devise the practice development plan (integrated evaluation, action and learning plan). When you are setting up the CCIs activities at this beginning stage, you will probably be interested in finding out:

1. The views that stakeholders hold about the setting/home and its care.
2. The experiences of care in the service/home that stakeholders have.
3. How they experience the climate/culture of the setting/home.
4. Their views on whether their experiences match up to the service's/ home's mission/philosophy.
5. Their views on the new vision statement.

As stated above, the CCIs evaluation tool can be used all the way through the practice development journey for a variety of purposes and by a variety of groups. So, the following guidance can be used at any stage.

You will need:

- approximately 15–30 minutes, depending on the size of the group;
- a flipchart easel, some flipchart paper and a pen;
- three differently coloured sets of sticky notes if you are doing Option B or creative arts materials for Option C.

Option A

Put up the three headings (Claims, Concerns, Issues) on a flipchart sheet. Invite group members/stakeholders to put forward their claims first, followed by their concerns. Ensure the suggestions from each person are all captured and not discussed or modified by other group members at this point. Give the group members an opportunity to add any final contributions. To identify the issues, the facilitator asks group members to identify any questions that can be developed from either the claims or concerns and that they want to see being taken forward.

Encourage **what** and **how** questions as these are the most useful in guiding action planning. For example, if the concern was about not always giving patients/residents choice in their day-to-day care or life, then the questions could be:

- What can we do to improve giving choices for patients/residents?
- How can we ensure that all team members are consistent in giving choice to people every day?

These questions help us to develop action plans about what we are going to do about giving choice and evaluation plans about how we are going to review that we are being consistent in giving choice.

Option B

This activity can also be done by inviting group members/stakeholders to write CCIs on sticky notes and put them onto three flipchart sheets that have been headed Claims, Concerns and Issues, respectively. Decide which colour sticky note is to be used for claims, which for concerns and which for issues. Any number of sticky notes can be used for each, but only one statement per note. Members put their statements on the appropriate flipchart sheets. The use of sticky notes enables theming to be more easily carried out if needed, as they can be moved around the flipchart sheet(s).

Option C

CCIs can also be expressed as artwork and then described by the creator. The key words are captured by the facilitator on the flipchart.

Follow-up work, coordinated by the practice development group, with all three options could include the items below.

- Share the CCIs from each group with all the other groups so that they can discuss similarities and differences with their CCIs. Generate as much agreement as possible.
- Ask the groups to make lists of the items about which there is no, or incomplete, agreement. Generate a combined list.
- Facilitate a discussion about how the items of the list will be taken forward into other sessions of CCIs with other stakeholders.
- Repeat the CCIs at an agreed future time and compare with the original one.
- As the practice development plan is carried out, CCIs can be carried out on any topic that arises during the plan's implementation.
- Sharing the CCIs with managers and other people in the organisation.

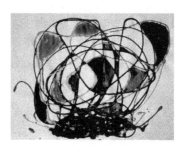

Chapter 5 Getting Started Together: Measuring and Evaluating Where We Are Now

Contents

Introduction

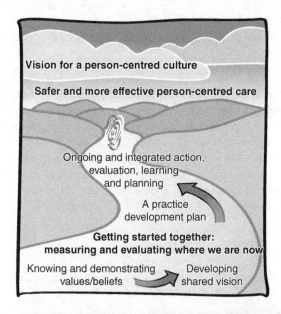

Fig. 5.1 The next step: Measuring and evaluating where we are now.

Vision for a person-centred culture

Safer and more effective person-centred care

Ongoing and integrated action, evaluation, learning and planning

A practice development plan

Getting started together: measuring and evaluating where we are now

Knowing and demonstrating values/beliefs

Developing shared vision

Chapter 5 builds on the introduction to measuring and evaluation in Chapter 4. In the first instance, the chapter is likely to be **useful to the group that has taken on the responsibility for planning the measuring and evaluating** of the baseline or where the workplace is now. The chapter will help this planning/coordinating group to explore which tools and methods they will recommend in the evaluation plan. Then the guides and tools will be **useful to those who volunteer or are asked to help carry out the**

Practice Development Workbook for Nursing, Health and Social Care Teams, First Edition. Jan Dewing, Brendan McCormack, and Angie Titchen.
© 2014 John Wiley & Sons, Ltd. Published 2014 by John Wiley & Sons, Ltd.
Companion website: www.wiley.com/go/practicedevelopment/workbook

evaluation. The role they play will vary according to people's capacity and desires. They may be involved in collecting, analysing or making sense of the evidence. Or they may provide evidence by telling their stories of giving or receiving care, for example. Please don't be put off by the number of tools and methods. No practice development work would ever use them all – you do not have to use them all. By offering choice, you will be able to find the tools or methods that best fit your evaluation questions, your setting and the people in it.

Getting started on the practice development journey towards the vision of person-centred care begins with measuring and evaluating the current situation, culture and care given in the workplace. As we introduced in Chapter 4, teams need to do this so that it becomes clearer what needs to be done in order to improve care. It is very similar to the idea of assessment for preparing a care plan. In Chapter 4, you were introduced to the importance of measuring and evaluation at the beginning of the implementation, as well as all the way through and at the end. You also worked with the idea that through learning, evaluation has the potential for making a contribution to many kinds of changes, for example changing your understanding about yourself and others. In practice development we refer to this as transformational change. We also talked about how systematic evaluation can improve collaboration, inclusion and participation of all stakeholders (those who have a stake in the change and will be affected by it) in bringing change about.

This chapter offers you a comprehensive framework for systematic evaluation that can integrate the processes of transformation along with achieving the evaluation outcomes. Evaluation outcomes are what the evidence (i.e. information or data) tells you, that is, a particular goal on your practice development journey has been achieved or you have reached the ultimate outcome of person-centred care. We also said that the evidence shows us how we are making progress. For example, it might demonstrate that we are working in more person-centred ways as we gather information and make sense of it. Or the evidence shows that we are learning to be more collaborative, inclusive and participative.

Before getting to the point of developing a comprehensive framework for systematic evaluation, the following phases (or something similar to these) will have taken place:

1. working out the shared values and beliefs and vision for the stakeholders and service;
2. converting the key purposes into vision statements;
3. using the vision statements to identify core evaluation questions and stakeholder Claims, Concerns and Issues to identify sub-questions;
4. identifying what evidence is already available and retrievable within the workplace/organisation/community.

In this chapter, we refer to a practice development coordinating group of key stakeholders that has been set up in the workplace to lead and coordinate the evaluation and the development of the action plans that emerge from it, as well as the implementation and evaluation of the practice development plan itself (see Chapter 6). Or an evaluation sub-group may have been set up. Such a coordinating group can ensure maximum efficiency, effectiveness and success of the practice development journey. However, if such a group hasn't been set up in your workplace, this chapter is still useful for you as an individual or if you are working with a group or groups of your co-workers and patients/residents to develop person-centred care.

The materials and tools in this chapter are organised around the following areas:

- setting up and running an effective practice development coordinating group;
- identifying stakeholders and developing a communication plan for how to best get their commitment;
- developing evaluation questions based on the vision statement;
- doing an analysis of the things in the workplace that could have a positive or negative influence on achieving the vision;
- methods for doing the evaluation;
- plans for learning from the evaluation.

Resources in this chapter

- **Guidance on developing evaluation questions** – this explains how to develop the evaluation questions from the Claims, Concerns and Issues (CCIs) (see Chapter 4) and how these questions will guide the gathering of evidence
- **Templates for analysing and recording positive and negative influences on achieving the vision in the workplace** – one tool is called a **S**trengths, **W**eaknesses, **O**pportunities and **T**hreats or SWOT analysis. The other tool is a Forcefield analysis that shows the relative degree of positive to negative influences in the workplace that

might impact on achieving the vision and the evaluation. These tools will help you to plan how to build on strengths to overcome weaknesses. Whilst they are useful to use at the beginning of the practice development journey, they can also be used for action planning about the various stages of the journey. These tools were previously published in Dewing & Titchen (2007).

- **Methods** – a wide range of methods are presented including posters, information sheets, consent forms, templates and guidance for collecting the evidence that is all around you in your setting through observations of care and the workplace, walkabouts, conversations, stories about patients/residents' and families' experiences. On the companion website, particular guidance is given for gaining consent from people with severe cognitive impairments, so that they can participate in the evaluation if they so wish. Methods for gathering evidence have been used by practice developers in the Irish practice development programme, *The Implementation of a Model of Person-Centred Practice in Older Person Settings* (McCormack et al., 2010) and at Cambridge University Hospitals NHS Foundation Trust (Dewing & Titchen, 2007). The methods set out here are an amalgam of our own experiences of working with them as well as those of other practice developers. Tools are also offered to measure person-centredness in the workplace, the climate or culture of the workplace or team. The analysis of the evidence gathered through these methods is presented in Chapter 6.

> In this resource, we often refer to, or give examples from, the Ireland practice development programme. Since the completion of that programme, the Health Service Executive (2010) has published a guide developed from the Irish programme, entitled *Enhancing Care for Older People – A Guide to Practice Development Processes to Support and Enhance Care in Residential Settings for Older People.* We recommend Sections 4 and 5 of the Ireland guide as complementary to this chapter here.
>
> You can access the complete programme report and a workplace learning resource from www.lenus.ie
>
> You may also find the Frequently Asked Questions relating to measuring and evaluating in Chapter 9 in this resource useful.

Guidance on developing evaluation questions

> This guidance is prepared primarily for a practice development coordinating group or its evaluation sub-group if it has one

To recap from Chapters 3 and 4, the overall purpose of the measuring and evaluation is first to show you where to go to achieve your vision statement and second, to find out whether you got there. Linked to this purpose are the evaluation questions that will act as your guide on the practice development journey. These questions are created from the vision statement. First, your questions will help you to become clear about what evidence you need to gather to see whether you have achieved your vision. Second, they will help you to pay attention to how you did it, so that you can learn about yourself and others and how to improve care in the future.

For example, key questions created from a vision statement about person-centred care might look something like this:

1. How can we create a culture in the workplace that is experienced as person-centred by all who work/live and visit here?
2. What is it like for patients/residents, staff and families during the culture change?
3. How will we know that we have achieved a person-centred culture?
4. How can we make our care of patients/residents and families more person-centred?
5. How can we make our working relationships with colleagues more person-centred?
6. What is it like for patients/residents, families and staff, during the change to make care more person-centred?
7. How will we know that we are delivering person-centred care?

The questions (issues) arising from the Claims, Concerns and Issues (CCIs) activities with stakeholders discussed in Chapter 4 can be discussed by the practice development coordinating group to see where those questions (issues) fit under the key evaluation questions. These sub-questions provide further guidance as stakeholders start out on measuring and evaluating.

SWOT or TOWS tool

This tool is for the practice development coordinating group or its evaluation sub-group if it has one

Once the group is clear about the evaluation questions, this tool and the next, adapted from Dewing & Titchen (2007), can be used to identify positive and negative factors in the workplace that you can build on or address in your evaluation plan and later in your practice development plan.

Strengths What do we do well? What are our strengths? What resources do we already have to draw on?	**Weaknesses** What do we do less well? What areas are not our strengths? What additional resources do we need to draw on?
Opportunities What opportunities can we capitalise on? What opportunities will we open up? How will we turn strengths into opportunities?	**Threats** What can harm our practice development? How do our weaknesses cause threats?

Forcefield analysis

This *tool can be used for any desired outcome, for example, achieving the vision statements and objectives. Here you could use it for your evaluation plan.*

Forcefield analysis: What factors may help or hinder the achievement of . . . our measuring and evaluation plan?

1. Identify your desired outcome (your objective).
2. Group members identify factors that may help them to achieve the plan (driving forces).
3. Group members identify factors that may hinder them in achieving the plan (restraining forces).
4. Each member considers each force and gives it a value (e.g. 0 = not relevant/no force, 1 = low force, 2 = medium force, 3 = high force).
5. Add up the score for each factor.
6. Factors with the most points need to receive the most attention.
7. Plan how to overcome the restraining forces and harness the driving forces to achieve your vision/objective.

Driving forces	Restraining forces

Gathering evidence in the workplace

This guidance is for the practice development coordinating group or its evaluation sub-group, if it has one, and staff, patients/residents, family members and volunteers who are going to help to collect the evidence

The evaluation questions that you have developed together with stakeholders through the CCIs activity can now guide you in thinking about what evidence you need to collect for the baseline. So for example, you may need to think about how you could collect evidence on the kind of culture in the workplace or, for example, the way patients/residents and staff are given or not given respect/freedom. Remember, there may already be evidence available in the workplace that you could use. There may be work done by individuals (and buddies) and in the small group discussions when using the activities in Chapter 2. For instance, in relation to the activities about values and beliefs, there might be notes and worksheets available (if people are prepared to share them) and the records of key points and action plans from the group discussions. Someone may also have done one or more rounds of the quick evaluation tool (available on the companion website) that is another source of evidence. In addition, there may be reports of a recent external audit or inspection done in the workplace that could be used. However it is likely that you will want to supplement this evidence with more in-depth observations of what goes on and hear patients/residents' and relatives' experiences. You might consider using tools as well, to measure person-centredness and the workplace or team cultures, for example. It would be worth browsing the companion website as there are tools there that might be useful.

But before you begin to collect evidence, it is important to ensure that patients, residents, families and staff in the workplace know what is going on, and are collaborating or participating in some way. This is where the coordinating group's communication plan with stakeholders is vital. You will need to check whether all the communications have been made and what support has been offered. It would be worth the group considering preparing some posters, a newsletter or information leaflets about the practice development evaluation to keep all stakeholders up-to-date with what is going on after their contributions to the vision statement.

If you are gathering evidence from people with a severe cognitive impairment, talking with them can sometimes be challenging and you will need to adapt your methods in some cases. This is especially so where the person has limited understanding of language or the ability to speak. So, the creative learning we've been showing you can come in very useful when thinking about ways in which you might get more involvement with patients/residents who have severe cognitive impairment.

For some of these people, it might simply be a case of ensuring that you have a bit more time and the environment is quiet. Then for others you may need to give clear written questions or use photos or objects to help the patient/resident connect with the topic you want to discuss. *Talking Mats* might be an idea you would like to consider (www.talkingmats.com).

Ten tips to help communication with people who have severe cognitive impairment

1. Always believe that communication in some way is possible.
2. Be a good listener; give the person your full attention and resist the temptation to finish what they are trying to say.
3. Talk at a slower pace so that the person has an opportunity to grasp what is being said.
4. Try to focus on the intention or positive aspects of what the person is saying and not the mistakes.
5. Read body language and gestures as well.
6. Avoid making assumptions; check things out with the person.
7. Avoid the use of jargon, multiple questions and complicated explanations.
8. Keep your conversation as simple as possible without being patronising
9. Avoid questions which have 'why' in them.
10. Say if you don't understand and ask the person to help you understand.

During evaluation and planning for the practice development, you may find the tips below helpful for involving and consulting people with severe cognitive impairment.

Tips for improving involvement and consultation with patients/residents who have severe cognitive impairment

- It is possible to consult patients/residents about their views of services.
- It is possible for staff to undertake service user consultation work.
- Staff need to be open-minded about approaches that seem unsuccessful.
- Documentation and reflection are important parts of the process.
- Particular approaches to communication may function as confidence-boosters for staff.
- Many patients/residents express needs and preferences in non-verbal ways.
- The issue of seeking consent applies to practice development.
- Communication and consultation can be personally very demanding for some persons with severe cognitive impairment.
- There is a need to recognise the importance of apparently small details of communication.
- Approaches to communication and consultation must be developed on an individual basis.
- Giving the person with severe cognitive impairment maximum control over opportunities for communication and, subsequently, consultation seems to be the best strategy.
- Devising and trying out approaches to communication and consultation requires time and energy.
- Communication and consultation should not be seen as a special activity that is set apart from other work.
- Investing effort in developing communication and so consultation can be highly rewarding for staff.
- Staff need to be helped to recognise the complexity of consultation and be prepared to learn new skills.
- There are limitations in adopting pre-planned approaches.

(Adapted from Allan, 2001)

We recommend that you take a look at the *Useful websites and resources* section at the end of this chapter.

> If you visit **www.wiley.com/go/practicedevelopment/workbook** you will find resources that will be helpful to you in planning for collecting evidence in your care setting, including:
>
> - a poster/flyer about gathering evidence;
> - a poster/information sheet about observations of practice;
> - an information sheet for families/decision makers of people for whom process consent might apply (e.g. people with severe cognitive impairment);
> - a guide to the method and documentation of the consent process for individuals with severely impaired capacity to consent to take part in a project;
> - person-centred assessment tools.

Giving and receiving feedback after evidence has been gathered

This guide is for team members, volunteers, patients/residents and family members who have agreed to participate with observations of care and the workplace

Giving and receiving feedback

If we are going to learn from our observations of care and the workplace, then as observers, we need to give others feedback about what we have observed. Communication of feedback needs to be based on openness and honesty. In turn, this means that we have to be able to offer clear and useful feedback to the people we work with and also to ensure that they can offer it to us. Preparing others including the team for receiving feedback and their role in making this a positive experience needs to start before data or evidence has been collected.

Think of times when you have been given feedback. What, in your experience, makes feedback useful? And, what kind of feedback is unhelpful? What could the other person have done differently? How could you have behaved differently?

Compare your experiences with the following themes and principles developed by nurses and practice developers at Cambridge University Hospitals NHS Foundation Trust (see Dewing & Titchen, 2007: 10–35).

We have put the next two resources onto separate pages in case you wish to copy them for use as posters or handouts.

Feedback is not criticism

Themes arising about **CRITICISM**	Themes arising about **FEEDBACK**
• lack of interpersonal skills in the giver is perceived as negative by receiver • has negative effects on the receiver • outcomes, e.g. destructive or unproductive • criticism when it's judgemental, i.e. making judgements about the value of something or of another's behaviour • focuses on the person • criticism is perceived as being harsh and disabling to the recipient • criticism looks like 'jumping in with both feet', i.e. hasn't been verified or checked out before talking • unstructured • problem-focused • focused on past or present	• enabling • positive, e.g. constructive and planned • specific skills for giving feedback • structured • supportive • positive effects on receiver • considered response • non-judgemental • action from positive outcomes • nature of feedback may be negative as well as positive • learning or solution focused • future oriented

Principles for giving and receiving feedback

1. Get the facts right before giving feedback.
2. Plan in advance how you are going to give feedback.
3. Prepare feedback carefully and practise.
4. Identify appropriate methods for giving feedback.
5. Encourage others involved to feel part of the process in advance so that it doesn't feel like a 'them and us' situation.
6. Work with the workplace manager or clinical leader so that she/he can help with the giving of feedback to others including staff.
7. Encourage recipients of feedback to take an opportunity to share their own self-assessment first before giving feedback from patient/resident narratives, e.g. asking 'What do you think patients/residents here are specifically saying about how they experience our service?'
8. Give support before, during and after giving feedback.
9. Give feedback on behaviour/issues not the person and their 'personhood' (i.e. be gentle with the person, firm on the behaviour/issues).
10. Enable increased self-awareness of behaviour and its consequences.
11. Provide non-judgemental feedback that is truthful, direct and constructive.
12. Focus on how the receiver of feedback can be in a position to move forward.
13. Provide follow-up.
14. Enable recipients to give us feedback on how we gave the feedback and how it could have been more effective.
15. Provide an opportunity to enable others to action-plan based on feedback and provide opportunities to identify how to share and celebrate good practices.

(Adapted for use in a variety of workplaces from Dewing & Titchen, 2007)

Workplace observations: Walkabout guide

This guide is for team members, volunteers, patients/residents and family members who have agreed to do workplace observations

In the Chapter 2 companion website materials, we introduced the idea of walkabouts (as a way of creating a scenario for informal group discussion). Walkabouts can also be used in a more focused way for gathering evidence about the workplace for evaluation. The focus of your observation comes, of course, from the evaluation questions that were identified by examining the issues/questions that arose in the stakeholders' *Claims, Concerns and Issues* and from the subsequent discussion and agreement about what evidence needs to be gathered. The shorter walkabout method described in Discussion trigger 2.5: Scenarios created by sensory walkabouts (see Chapter 2 material on the companion website) can be used or the more focused approach described below.

As you are observing the workplace and not patients/residents or care workers, you do not need to gain formal written consent, but it is essential to get verbal consent. It is also good publicity for the practice development work to explain how the observations will be used to develop the practice development plan.

> For example, you might say something like this: 'Good afternoon, we are engaged in working together to make the unit/ward/clinic/care home more person-centred. Here is a poster showing this idea. Well, we are here today for a short time to capture what is going on in the communal areas. This will help us see whether we need to change anything. We won't be long. Is that OK? If not, we can come back later.'

If there are patients/residents in the shared space where you want to do the walkabout explain why you are there in ways that they can grasp. Also, if you don't know these people, find out from the care staff how you would recognise that your observations might be upsetting them (by their behaviour, expression or sounds, for example).

If you observe that anyone becomes unwell or distressed by your observations, you should end your observations in that space and ensure that the care team knows that the person is unwell/upset.

It is important to give feedback about your observation to the team members who are working in the *unit/ward/clinic/care home* during the observation period. It is vital to learn how to give feedback that is experienced by the person hearing it as a learning opportunity, rather than as criticism or a reprimand.

Preparation

- Ensure that you have read and reflected on the activities in 'Giving and receiving feedback after evidence has been gathered'.
- Organise a co-observer if you can as it is good to have more than one view.
- Meet with the workplace manager/clinical leader to discuss the purpose, process and expected outcomes of the observation and get her/his support for helping the team to carry out action plans that arise from the observations.
- Agree times and dates when observations will be carried out with the practice development coordinating group and discuss with them what will happen to the evidence and what is the time-scale.
- Negotiate these dates and times with the team members on duty.
- Ensure that all team members have given verbal consent for being observed (check the communication plan to see who was responsible for this if it wasn't you and find out whether verbal consent has been given).
- Consider consent issues by reading the Chapter 5 companion website material (**www.wiley.com/go/ practicedevelopment/workbook**)

You will need:

- 1 hour;
- your buddy or colleague;
- a copy of this sheet of instructions;
- a pen and a small notebook or piece of paper;
- two copies of the observation and action planning record sheets (one for you each) (see later in this section);
- the combined observation sheet for feedback to staff;
- someone who has agreed to support the team after the observation to help them learn from it.

Key activities

Meet the team leader or coordinator to check that the observation can go ahead as planned and that all the team on duty have given verbal consent. Explain that observing will take 30 minutes, preparing for giving feedback will take about 15 minutes and giving it to staff another 15 minutes.

Go to the front entrance of the workplace and pause for a moment or two before you go in to take a few deep breaths. As you go in together and walk about the public spaces in the workplace, use all your body senses to take the place in. Try to experience things with eyes and ears etc. wide open. As you come into the workplace, what do you see/hear/smell/touch/taste?

As you pause for a moment and then continue walking, notice how you feel about what you are seeing, hearing, smelling etc. Write down briefly (a word, phrases or images) or sketch roughly your observations and insights on your *Workplace observations record sheet*.

Keep focusing on your senses for the remaining time.

After 25 minutes, sit down with your buddy/colleague somewhere private and reflect on your observations. Ask yourself/yourselves:

- What do you notice that you have never noticed before? Why was that?
- Did anything shock or surprise you?
- What did your observations tell you about the workplace and, if there are any, the experience of patients/residents being here? (5–10 mins)

Agree between you the key observations and insights that came and record them on the *Combined observations: Record sheet for feedback*. Then discuss what and how you are going to feed these observations back to the staff who are on duty that day.

Give the feedback to as many of the team as possible in a quiet area, bearing in mind the principles for giving helpful feedback that we have already introduced in this section. The feedback should be structured around Sights, Sounds, Smells, Tastes and Touch. Consider:

- what I saw, heard, smelt, touched, felt, where, when and who;
- privacy, dignity and respect in the way you talk;
- opportunities for clarification by the team.

Record on the combined sheet any actions that the team, having heard your feedback, think they could take and who they are going to discuss their action plans with and get support from.

Date and sign the *Combined observations: Record sheet for feedback* and photocopy it. Keep one copy, give others to the team members working during the observation and another to the person who has agreed to provide support for the team members.

The original should be given to the practice development coordinating group or evaluation sub-group who will look at all the observations and use them to feed into the practice development plan. At that stage, the group will agree a set of actions that they would propose to the manager/clinical leader. They would also agree who would meet with the manager/clinical leader and consider what they wanted to achieve and a plan of how they would discuss this with the manager/clinical leader. The agreed actions with the manager/clinical leader would then get fed into the practice development plan. This coordinated approach prevents all kinds of 'random' actions being undertaken and chaos resulting!

The group will also ensure safe storage of the evidence.

Repeat the observations at intervals agreed in the practice development plan (see Chapter 6) and give feedback as above. As you feel more confident in doing this activity you can begin to facilitate other team members to join in. Observation of their own workplace and practice by team members, students and other learners is a very powerful learning activity and one that is encouraged within practice development.

This guide can also be used to do the quick evaluation (available on companion website).

Workplace observations: In a fixed place

> This guide is for team members, volunteers, patients/residents and family members who have agreed to participate with workplace observations

Another way to carry out workplace observations in shared spaces in the workplace is for you and your buddy/colleague to position yourself, unobtrusively, in a fixed spot, for the whole 30 minute observation period, and for observations to be carried out at different times of day. The Workplace Walkabout guide above can be used. The only difference is that you are not walking about!

Workplace observations: Record sheet

Date of observation: _____   Done by: _____

Observation	Insight

Names of team members who have given verbal consent for observation are:

_____

_____

_____

_____

_____

Combined observations: Record sheet for feedback

Date: Done by:

Key observations	Insights	Action to be taken

Guide: Observations of care

This guide is for team members who have agreed to participate with observations of care

Observing care giving is very sensitive and a great deal of thought should be given that patients/residents are comfortable with you being there, even if they have already given you consent. The care worker(s) you are observing know the patient/resident so you should ask them to tell you if the patient/resident is getting distressed (when you don't pick it up), and the observation should be ended immediately.

For observations of the care of patients/residents follow the guide for the workplace observations, but in addition, take very special care that you are sure that the person with severe cognitive impairment has also been offered the opportunity to give their consent – in whatever way they do this. Although some people may not be able to give informed consent they can still communicate their choices and preferences. This form of consent giving is based on how things feel rather than on what the person thinks about them; it is known as process consent (Dewing 2007, 2008b, 2009b). See the information sheet for families/decision-makers and the guide for the method and documentation for process consent (available on companion website).

You will need to negotiate with care team members whether you follow them around for a 30 minute period as they care for people or whether you stay with one particular person receiving care (and relative or friend if present) and observe the care given by whoever comes into the area/room in the 30 minute period.

If you and your buddy observe anything that worries you, for example you feel that a member of the team is upsetting someone then, as a fellow worker, indicate at the time that you are worried, perhaps by saying 'I think Fred is getting a bit upset, would it be best to leave that for now?' When you feed back the combined observations, tell them why you were concerned and ask them whether they would like some support from the person who has agreed to give support should the staff want it. Other examples might be that lunch is left uneaten and no one appears to have noticed, or the toilet door is open when the toilet is being used. The thing is not to blame or be judgemental, but to point things out to help the team members to become more aware so that they can take the action that is needed.

Guide: Patient/resident/relative narrative interview

This guide is for team members, volunteers, patients/residents or family members who have agreed to do narrative interviews

Preparation for you   Narrative interviews are conversations loosely guided by a number of questions prepared in advance. These questions are merely prompts to help the person being interviewed to talk about their experiences. Some examples of guiding questions are given below.

Interviews are usually done by one person so that the patient/resident/relative/friend does not feel anxious or overwhelmed by having two or more people listening to what they say. It is important, therefore, that you learn how to do an interview before you have a go. You could do this by working with your learning buddy in a mock interview, following all the guidance below with the modification that you will be interviewing them about their experience of working in the setting. So you could ask, for example, 'Can you describe being a member of the care team here?' or 'What is it like being a care worker here?' You should also practise taking notes during the interview. When you have finished, ask your buddy to give you feedback on how it felt being interviewed by you. Both of you need to be familiar with giving and receiving feedback constructively.

In advance, you should also check whether an information flyer about the evaluation has been made in the workplace for giving to the person you are hoping to interview. If not, you could prepare one and then share it with other co-workers to get their feedback on it and for them to use in their interviews.

Preparation for the patient/resident/relative/friend   When you are confident to do an interview with a patient/resident, relative or friend, you should seek permission before you conduct the interview preferably 24 hours before, so that when the appointed time comes, they can be really sure that they want to take part or have thought of any further questions for clarification. The exception to this is where the person has severe cognitive impairment where, when legal capacity is lacking, you will need to use the process consent method (see companion website). Here you will need to discuss consent and begin the interview together.

If you are interviewing, you should give patients/residents the opportunity to have a relative or friend there to support them and help them to say what they want to say. If they want this, you should be clear to them and the relative or friend, that it is the patient/resident's views that you are seeking and not the relative's or friend's views. If the relative or friend would like their views heard then you would arrange a separate interview for them (at which the patient/ resident could be there in the support role if they wanted to).

First, you need to provide the patient/resident/relative/friend with information on the purpose of the interview, that is, that their experiences will be used to help improve person-centred care in the workplace. You should offer the information leaflet at this time. Stress that whatever they say will be confidential. You should also tell them that you will be feeding back their experiences anonymously to the care team to help them to improve their care. You should assure them that no one is going to get into 'trouble' because of what you say, because the intent is to improve and not to blame. Adapt this process for patients/residents with severe cognitive impairments.

Show that you will take notes of what they say and that, if desired, you will show them the notes afterwards to check for accuracy. You should also say that they are free to stop the interview at any time and that this will not be held against them or affect their or their relative/friend's care adversely in any way. You should give them an opportunity to ask any questions about the purpose of the interview and what will happen. By doing all this in advance, you can also ask the patient/resident whether they would like their relative or friend to be with them during the interview to support them.

You must always obtain permission from the person before actually starting the interview, so you need to repeat the above information if they are still not clear what you are asking their permission for.

When seeking and obtaining consent from people with severe cognitive impairment, it may be necessary to do this in a different way, especially if they have advanced severe cognitive impairment. Therefore, a separate guide is provided in the next resource.

Doing the unstructured interview (30 minutes or less)

The time the interview will take depends on how the patient/resident/relative/friend is feeling but also on how much time you have. Try to have 30 minutes, but be sensitive to the person's needs.

To really get at individuals' experiences, it is important not to put words into their mouths. Therefore the way you ask questions is really important. Your questions should be open to invite the person to expand and should not lead the person to respond in any particular way. Rather the questions are to help them tell you whatever is important to them and what they think might improve the care and service provided by the workplace. Avoid closed questions that only invite Yes/No answers as these responses are less useful.

Examples of guiding questions

1. Start by using an opening question such as 'How are you today?' The answer to this may or may not be used in the narrative analysis.
2. What is it like to be a patient/resident/relative/friend here?
3. What was life like when you were younger?
4. What idea or plans do you have for the future?
5. How do you spend your days here? Or: describe your day to me.
6. Do you have any ideas for improvements in the workplace or for improving patients/residents' experiences?
7. Is there anything else you would like to tell me about your experience/life here?

Guide: Conversation with patients/residents with severe cognitive impairment

This guide is for team members, volunteers or family members who have agreed to have a conversation with a patient/resident with a severe cognitive impairment

If doing an interview with a patient/resident with a severe cognitive impairment is not the best way to find out what it is like for them in the workplace because direct questioning is too cognitively demanding or meaningless for them, then it may be better to communicate in the way that they naturally interact with others. So, for example, if a person likes to wander-walk around the workplace or garden and chat to those they meet, then you might ask them if you can accompany them on their walk for 30 minutes or so. You might strike up a conversation with them then by following their lead with whatever they want to say or express at that moment. In this more informal way than an interview, you can try to get a sense of what life is like for them. For example, for a person who likes to wander-walk outside, finding the garden door locked causes them frustration or finding it open gives them pleasure. You could then ask them how they are feeling at that moment and go wherever the conversation takes you. Taking the person away into a quiet room to talk probably won't work very well, as neither of you will have environmental cues to draw on in your conversation.

Providing information about the purpose of the conversation and for getting their consent should be done in a way that persons with severe cognitive impairment can grasp. For instance, you might show photos about what you want to chat about and show the person that you are going to write or draw a few things in your notebook. You could encourage them to touch the notebook and look inside if they want to. If you don't know the person with severe cognitive impairment, then ask their carer, relative or friend how you can best communicate with them and how you would know that they are happy for you to begin or continue with a conversation. You should also find out how the person shows that they are fine or upset by their use of certain behaviours, expressions, gestures, sounds and so on. If you see any signs that suggest that they are distressed, you should stop the conversation, provide support and let the carer know the situation.

See the documentation for process consent earlier in this chapter, as this may give you ideas for what you need to check out.

The communication tips offered earlier in this chapter about asking questions can also be useful as a reminder for you:

- Avoid asking 'why' questions.
- Ask clear simple questions such as – what is this place like?
- Try to make statements first, such as, some people being looked after/living here feel . . . what about you?
- Listen very carefully and give the extra time that you feel is needed.

By the way, working like this is very person-centred as it responds to the patient/resident with severe cognitive impairment in a way that suits them. So gathering evidence like this might also be a learning opportunity for you.

Team culture tool (Pritchard & Dewing, 2000)

This guide is for the workplace team including care staff, housekeeping staff and the manager/clinical leader to assess the culture in the team. The team might decide to analyse the results themselves. They could use the results to inform plans for workplace culture change that will support person-centred care. The workplace team might also be interested in participating in a workshop on workplace culture. Our experience of facilitating this workshop with large numbers of people over the last decade or more is that it is a really good investment of time in terms of the impact it has on people and the subsequent changes they make. Guidance on facilitating this workshop can be found in the companion website.

Think about the culture of **YOUR TEAM**. Your team could be the people you work with in the workplace. Read through the list (a to l) below and circle the number on each question that identifies the nearest to where you think **YOUR TEAM** is.

EXAMPLE

People in my team break rank and go it alone	1	2	3	4	5	People in my team pull together

If I circle 1, then I feel my team work on their own most of the time. If I circle 3, I think they work alone some of the time and pull together as a team some of the time. If I circle 5, I feel that on the whole my team works together. This questionnaire should take **5–15 minutes** to complete.

a) People in my team have dissimilar values, interests and beliefs	1	2	3	4	5	People in my team share values, interests and beliefs
b) People in my team break rank and go it alone	1	2	3	4	5	People in my team pull together
c) Individuals in my team operate alone and there is conflict between them	1	2	3	4	5	There is community spirit and co-operation in my team
d) My team is ruled by standards of the past	1	2	3	4	5	My team is ruled by visions of the future
e) Meetings are an aspect of the culture in my team	1	2	3	4	5	Working in small teams is an aspect of the culture in my team
f) In my team there are winners and losers, them and us	1	2	3	4	5	People confront and move beyond their differences in my team
g) My team is anti-change	1	2	3	4	5	My team is change oriented
h) There is weak coordination in my team	1	2	3	4	5	There is strong coordination in my team
i) My team is inward-looking and is focused on itself	1	2	3	4	5	My team is outward-looking and does not focus on itself
j) My team is dominated by routine and systems	1	2	3	4	5	My team is creative and ideas-dominated
k) People do not reflect about their work in my team	1	2	3	4	5	People reflect about their work in my team
l) There is disagreement in my team	1	2	3	4	5	There is harmony in my team

Thank you for completing this questionnaire.

Making sense of the results When you look at the results, scores that are closer to 5 indicate a team that has shared values, a sense of openness, willingness to learn and is future focused – this is an integrated team. Look out for results that stand out either because they are high (close to 5) or low (closer to 1). Teams with low scores tend to be segmented. *See the next resource, a handout on these two types of teams and cultures. You can use this handout to trigger discussions.*

You may also get widely differing responses to the same question from different members. This can be because there is inconsistency in the team – so some members feel it is great and others feel it is pretty awful.

The results can be plotted on lines from 1–5 for each question so that a visual feedback can be offered.

If the results seem overly positive and this does not represent peoples' lived experiences, then a discussion can be had about why team members have offered the responses they have.

The aim is for the team to learn more about how members experience the team and what needs to be done to move forward.

Useful facilitative questions that are also solution and future focused can include:

On a scale of 0–5 where 5 equals us at our very best, where are we now?

What needs to happen for us to go on progressing up the scale?

What will you be doing differently at the next step up?

How will you (or significant others) be able to tell . . .?

Let's suppose that we get to the next step up tomorrow. What's the smallest sign that will tell you that things are improving?

What else?

What else?

What have we each done that's made it work this well?

What would you like to see yourself doing differently between now and next time we meet?

What needs to be different to make it even better?

What will you take away with you from this conversation?

Handout: Culture (Bate, 1995)

A culture can be defined as the way we do things around here (Drennan, 1992). This handout can be used by team members and volunteers to discuss whether they think the culture in the workplace is most like a segmentalist (fragmented) or an integrative (transformational) culture. A transformational culture supports transformation of people, teams, practices, services, workplaces and organisations.

The conclusions of your discussion can be recorded as evaluation evidence. If you were to tick the bullet points that are closest to your culture, it is likely that there will be ticks in both columns. It would be interesting to count the ticks in each column and then repeat the discussion in the team, say, a year later and see whether the ticks are moving to the right. (The most desirable culture is an integrative culture.)

SEGMENTALIST CULTURE	INTEGRATIVE CULTURE
• Disparate values, interests and beliefs	• Shared values, interests and beliefs
• Breaking rank, going it alone	• Pulling together
• Tribalism and conflict	• Communitas and co-operation
• Compartmentalising problems	• Seeing problems as wholes
• Ruled by standards of the past	• Ruled by visions of the future
• Meetings	• Teams
• Winners and losers / them and us	• Confronting and transcending differences
• Anti-change/reactionary	• Change-orientated
• Weak coordinating mechanism and lateral linkages	• Strong coordination mechanisms and lateral linkages
• Inward-looking	• Outward-looking
• Mechanistic, systems-dominated	• Creative, ideas-dominated
• Non-reflective	• Reflective
• Discordant	• Harmonious

My notes: Comments and questions I have

Handout: Effective workplace culture (Manley et al. 2011)

> This handout can be used by facilitators in the workshop on workplace culture as described on the companion website. Alternatively, it can be used by a new facilitator as a discussion checklist to promote dialogue amongst the team, volunteers, patients/residents and family members about the current workplace culture.

The facilitator helps a group discuss whether they think the workplace culture has in place any of the enabling factors (things that help a culture to be effective), attributes (features) or consequences (outcomes of having such a culture). Conclusions of the discussion can be recorded as evaluation evidence. If you were to tick the things that everyone agrees are already in place, this record is kept safely as well. The discussion could be repeated a year later, then 2 years later to see whether there have been any changes and whether any more ticks can be added. Please note, it usually takes about 2 years for big cultural changes to take place, although small changes can be seen in just a few months. For example, in the short-term, you might hear staff no longer using de-personalising language like 'feeding' or 'doing the washes' and hear person-centred language like 'helping Mrs Brown to eat/wash'. Outcomes like individual, team and organisational effectiveness take longer.

| Effective[a] workplace culture[b] concept analysis |||
| Manley et al. (2011) (Reproduced by kind permission of the *International Practice Development Journal*) |||
Enabling factors	**Essential attributes**	**Consequences**

INDIVIDUAL:
• transformational leadership
• skilled facilitation
• role clarification.
ORGANISATIONAL:
• flattened and transparent management
• organisational readiness
• human resource management support.
	1. Specific values promoted in the workplace, namely:
	  • person-centredness
	  • lifelong learning
	  • support and challenge
	  • leadership development
	  • involvement, collaboration and participation by stakeholders (including service users)
	  • evidence-use and development
	  • positive attitude to change
	  • open communication
	  • teamwork
	  • safety (holistic).
	2. All the above values are realised in practice, there is a shared vision and mission and individual and collective responsibility.
	3. Adaptability, innovation and creativity maintain workplace effectiveness.
	4. Appropriate change is driven by the needs of patients/users/communities
	5. Formal systems (structures and processes) exist to continuously enable continuous evaluation of learning, evaluation of performance and shared governance[c].
		1. Continuous evidence that:
		  • Patients', users' and communities' needs are met in a person-centred way.
		  • Staff are empowered and committed.
		  • Standards and goals are met (individual, team and organisational effectiveness).
		  • Knowledge/evidence is developed, used and shared.
		2. Human flourishing for all.
		3. Positive influence on other workplace cultures.

[a] Effective = achieving the outcomes of person-centredness and evidenced-based care (performance).

[b] Workplace culture = the most immediate culture experienced and/or perceived by staff, patients, users and other key stakeholders. This is the culture that impacts directly on the delivery of care. It both influences and is influenced by the organisational and corporate culture as well as other idiocultures. Idioculture is used to imply that there are different cultures that exert an influence on each other rather than one organisational/corporate culture with sub-cultures within a hierarchical arrangement.

[c] Shared governance encompasses achieving stakeholder participation in using evidence from a variety of sources (e.g. audit, feedback, reflective practice, research) for decision making.

Useful websites and resources

For ease of use, this section is also available on the companion website: **www.wiley.com/go/practicedevelopment/ workbook**

The Productive Series

www.institute.nhs.uk/quality_and_value/productivity_series/the_productive_series.html

A presentation on Putting Patients First (www.institute.nhs.uk/images/documents/Productives/Putting%20 patients%20first%20-%20The%20Productive%20Series%20FINAL.pdf).

The following link takes you to a description about a Patient-Centred Care Project that drew on an approach called experience-based co-design (EBCD). This project aimed to improve the experience and quality of care for patients receiving treatment for breast cancer and lung cancer (www.kingsfund.org.uk/current_projects/point_of_care/ebcd_ evaluation.html).

With the right support, people living with dementia can express opinions about services. This report of a study explored how staff can encourage people with dementia to express their views and preferences in the course of day-to-day practice. Allan (2001) (www.jrf.org.uk/bookshop/eBooks/186134810X.pdf; www.jrf.org.uk/publications/ exploring-ways-staff-consult-people-with-dementia-about-services).

Talking Mats might be an idea you would like to consider (www.talkingmats.com). A project found that Talking Mats can be used by many people with dementia and that it improves their ability to communicate. The report suggests that Talking Mats can provide family and staff with a tool to enable many people with dementia to communicate their needs and preferences more easily than through usual conversation (www.jrf.org.uk/publications/ using-talking-mats-help-people-with-dementia-communicate).

Augmentative and Alternative Communication (AAC) covers a wide range of techniques to support or replace spoken communication. This website offers examples of low and high-tech methods, including gesture, signing, symbols, word boards, communication boards and books, as well as Voice Output Communication Aids (VOCAs) (www.communicationmatters.org.uk/page/talking-mats).

The Online Evaluation Resource Library (OERL) for education. This library was developed for professionals seeking to design, conduct, document or review project evaluations (http://oerl.sri.com/te.html).

OTseeker is a database that contains abstracts of systematic reviews and randomised controlled trials relevant to occupational therapy. Trials have been critically appraised and rated to assist you to evaluate their validity and interpretability. These ratings will help you to judge the quality and usefulness of trials for informing clinical interventions (www.otseeker.com).

Chapter 6 A Practice Development Plan

Contents

Introduction

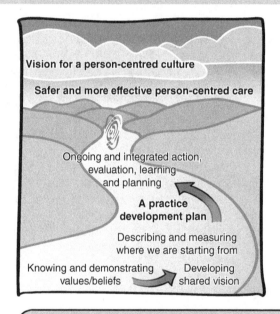

Fig. 6.1 The next step: A practice development plan for integrated action, learning and evaluation.

Chapter 6 is for those leading, coordinating and facilitating the development of practice. If you are in a practice development coordinating group or evaluation sub-group, this chapter is relevant for you. The guidance will help you to involve, and/or work with, staff, patients/residents and families to make a plan together for developing practice. You can make this happen by engaging people in the activities in this chapter. These activities are conducted with individuals, small informal groups and larger, formal groups. You may find the templates we offer on the companion website useful for making the plan.

Team members who are leading mini-projects (see Chapter 7), students and other learners (see Chapter 8) may also find the materials in here helpful.

You may also want to take a look at or have to hand two chapters from the book *Practice Development in Nursing and Healthcare* (McCormack et al., 2013) that are helpful in understanding the broader context of evidence in practice development and in seeing how person-centred practice can be evaluated. In Chapter 7, Jo Rycroft-Malone presents an overview of the PARIHS Framework – a framework for systematically guiding the use of evidence in practice. In Chapter 10, Brendan McCormack, Tanya McCance and Jill Maben discuss how person-centred practice outcomes can be evaluated.

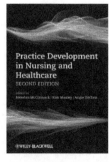

Practice Development Workbook for Nursing, Health and Social Care Teams, First Edition. Jan Dewing, Brendan McCormack, and Angie Titchen.
© 2014 John Wiley & Sons, Ltd. Published 2014 by John Wiley & Sons, Ltd.
Companion website: www.wiley.com/go/practicedevelopment/workbook

As in Chapter 5, we refer to a practice development coordinating group or an evaluation sub-group of key stakeholders set up in the care setting/care home to lead and coordinate the evaluation. The evaluation evidence will help the coordinating group (or those taking a lead, coordinating or facilitating role) in the care setting/care home to develop the practice development plan. It is helpful if this group or these people also coordinate the carrying out of the plan and evaluation of progress. Having such a group can ensure maximum efficiency, effectiveness and success of the development.

Clarifying values and beliefs, visioning and evaluating your starting point are vital processes for getting practice development going. However, there comes a point when a written practice development plan or action plan is required. The plan is a practical tool or guide to organise the actual implementation, the learning and the ongoing evaluation work that needs to take place. It's also something that all leaders and managers like to or need to have for reporting on quality improvement and innovation initiatives and projects. Before getting to the point of writing an action plan, the following phases (or something similar to these) will have taken place:

1. Working out the shared values and beliefs and vision for the stakeholders and service/home.
2. Converting the key purposes into vision statements.
3. Using the vision statements to identify core evaluation questions and stakeholder Claims, Concerns and Issues to identify sub-questions.
4. Identifying what evidence is already available that applies locally and is retrievable within the care setting/care home.
5. Identifying what evidence is not available or retrievable within the care setting/care home and how you will gather it.
6. Collating available evidence and gathering new evidence.
7. Prioritising to form a practice development plan.
8. Knowing what other plans exist in your care setting/care home and/or organisation to link work up together.
9. Creating an integrated evaluation, action and learning plan, i.e. a practice development plan.

Before introducing this section, a few words about developing action plans in larger organisations – Any new action plans must weave in with existing plans developed in the organisation. In particular, plans should fit with the aims and objectives of larger plans – for example, a quality improvement or governance plan will often be concerned with the same or similar aspects of care delivery that you are exploring here. Remember to find out what already exists and build on the good work of others that has already been started.

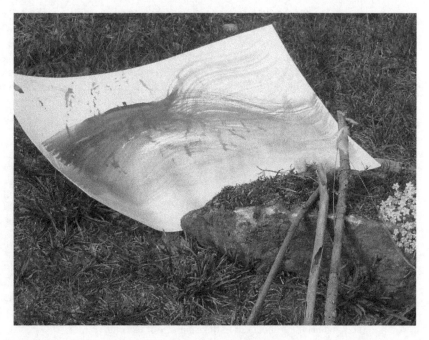

Fig. 6.2 Inviting people to paint what matters to them about the shared journey to be undertaken can free people up for action planning.

This chapter will help you and patients/residents and families prioritise what needs to go into the plan.

For example, in a special care baby unit, the team had decided to use the team culture tool (see Chapter 5) and were shocked to find that they scored lowly, indicating that they have a segmented culture in their team, rather than the desirable integrated team. They followed this up by organising a workshop on the culture (see companion website) in the unit. They invited parents, visitors and volunteers to join them at the workshop. Worryingly, the collages that this wider stakeholder group created also showed that very different values, interests and beliefs were rife in the unit. This was shown as people going off in their own directions without reference to others. In addition, the creative expressions showed in startlingly graphic ways that tribalism and conflict was tangible and that it was having very negative effects on the parents whose babies they were caring for. At the end of the workshop, all stakeholders agreed that although some of the attributes of an effective workplace culture (see Chapter 5), like safety and formal evaluation structures and processes, were in place, some other attributes were far from apparent at this current time. All present agreed that working together to transform the culture in the unit was crucial. They identified a number of things that should go into the practice development plan, such as a parent and team member doing a walkabout observation around the unit and feeding back to the team members on duty what they had seen, heard, felt and imagined. They also prioritised the need for team members to form an active learning group where they could challenge and support each other in changing the way they worked as a team.

Nursing team members in a surgical ward gathered narratives from patients about their experience of their post-op care after major surgery resulting in a stoma. When they analysed the stories they found that, on the whole, patients said that staff did not spend enough time with them helping them to develop knowledge and skill about how to look after their own stoma. For example, according to many of the patients, the nurses said that they didn't have time to do this and anyway, it was the job of the clinical nurse specialists to do the educa-tion. Their job was to change the bag and clean the stoma. Patients said that these behaviours and, in a few cases, barely disguised disgust when changing colostomy bags that had been left too long, not only prevented them from becoming independent in stoma self-care whilst they were in the ward, it also made them feel under-valued and rejected by health-care professionals. A few weeks later, when the team came together with the clinical nurse specialist, they invited previous patients (who were returning to the hospital that day for a 3 month check-up clinic that day) to attend a session to discuss ways that care could be improved on the ward.

The team had asked the clinical nurse specialist to facilitate the session as she had experience of working with groups and in creating safe spaces and conditions for conversations that could be honest, open and without blame or judgement. After presenting the key messages from the stories, the team asked the five patients present what sort of support they got and what they thought would have been helpful to them after their surgery some 3 months previously. The team listened respectfully and non-defensively and ideas were written up on a flipchart for everyone to see. At the end of the session, it was agreed that the notes and the plan to set up a practice development coordination group would be written up and circulated to those present if they so wished. It was agreed that this group would consider the ideas put forward at the session along with other evaluation data and come up with a draft action plan for discussion with stakeholders. Two of the patients present offered to join the coordinating group and they were warmly thanked by the team.

In another example, at High Downs Care Home, the team have found out from their observations and from older peoples' narratives that meals are rushed and focused on the team getting through the tasks of serving and clearing away the food, rather than on the social and pleasurable aspects of eating together. This team's first actions could then centre around raising awareness of this issue in the home and working with patients/residents and those who serve meals to make plans about how to make eating in the dining room more homely and sociable.

Next the team has to agree HOW they will go about doing this, WHO will be helping and by WHEN they will achieve their actions. They can also explain WHY the action plan is needed to others in the home.

Also, as decisions about actions are made with relevant stakeholders, we offer you some ideas in this section about how you might go about this partnership way of working.

Regardless of how good practice development plans (alternatively called action plans) are in themselves, there are many obstacles in the care setting/care home context as well as inside ourselves that prevent the agreed or required action actually happening. You may have identified some of these obstacles if you did the SWOT analysis or Forcefield analysis in Chapter 5, and there will be more opportunities to do so here if you didn't. Recognition of obstacles is needed to ensure practice developers know what lies ahead, and can therefore plan how they will address or reduce the significance of them. It is also important that the processes used within action plans are consistent with the shared values and beliefs and agreed processes or ways of working (see Chapter 3).

An action plan is a list of activities and/or tasks that a practice development group or stakeholders have to carry out to move towards the practice development vision in a planned and systematic way. It differs from an action list or 'to do' list in that it focuses on the achievement of one rather than several goals. It also has stages or steps for the activities (sequencing), timescales, named responsibility, necessary resources and support, possibly core, active and peripheral stakeholders and finally criteria for success evaluation.

Action plans are likely to be about what changes are to be made but also about what has to be learned to make the changes and how that can be facilitated. Based on the findings from a study about the implementation of a model of person-centred practice (Dewing et al., 2007), the main learning areas for your care setting/care home might be about:

1. **decision-making** – a movement from top down, controlled decision-making to decision-making in which the team and patients/residents participate is needed to evolve person-centred cultures. Care staff can develop joint decision making with patients/residents and management.
2. **relationships** – changing relationships from those rooted in roles and responsibilities (that are often draining on both personal and team energy) to those that are based in working together in partnership, generates energy for new ideas, growth and development.
3. **resolving conflictual ways of working** – rather than engaging in negative and destructive ways of working, a range of forums and other opportunities such as practice development working groups, generating new ideas and learning from practice can be nurtured. To achieve this, team members need skills for critical reflection, problem solving, solution-focused dialogues and working collaboratively with a range of stakeholders.
4. **application or use of power** – a power shift from the traditional 'power over others' approach to power as a resource to enable others to learn, grow and develop can help practice development and also create a nicer atmosphere, which can be 'felt' by staff, patients/residents, families and visitors.
5. **processes for learning** – encouraging eagerness to learn and translating this into action, and enabling similar learning in others, can help widen the impact of practice development in the workplace.

Action planning is a necessary activity for achieving and monitoring changes in practice and service delivery, so it will be vital that the plan shows how it relates to any broader strategy your care setting/care home has for service delivery and/or organisational development.

Resources in this chapter

- **Pulling it together** – guidelines for analysing evidence, checking out the analyses with stakeholders and comparing evidence from different sources and agreeing what matters and should be prioritised. A two-part series of individual and small, informal group activities and a three-part series of formal workshops offer alternative ways of preparing for action planning and prioritisation. The group activities are shorter and less comprehensive than the workshops, so if time is tight, you might choose the activities over the more systematic workshops. The activities and workshops are grouped according to their purpose, so that you can see them side by side to make your choice easier between activity or workshop or a mix of the two.
- **Person-centred care template** – in which you can set out your starting point of your practice development journey from the findings from your evaluation evidence. The template also shows the end point of your practice development journey. Having a clearer idea of your starting and end points will help you to plan how you are going to get to the end point and achieve your vision. Filled in templates are offered to show you how you can use them to map your journey and to inspire you.
- **Action planning** – this includes a detailed overview action planning guide and template that the practice development group and other small groups of stakeholders might find useful.
- **Action point planning sheet** (available on companion website) – this is a very simple sheet that helps you and participants at meetings and workshops keep hold of action points so they are not lost over the course of the meeting. It also provides a format for ensuring that when action points are agreed, timescales and named persons take ownership for carrying out the action. More complex actions, or actions where obstacles are likely to be encountered, may need more in-depth action plans, such as those offered in this Chapter.

- **SMART and SMARTER goals handout** – this handout can be used as a resource in facilitating discussions about goal setting in practice development work. Using the tool as a template can enable practitioners to have a practice or trial run through possible goals or milestones (as they also need to be SMART or SMARTER).

In Chapter 9, there are Frequently Asked Questions that may be helpful *when you get going on developing the practice development plan.*

Pulling it together activity 1: Individual/informal group activity for analysis of evidence (in preparation for action planning)

This short activity (Activity 1) and the next longer, more systematic and comprehensive workshop 1, are about analysing evidence. Activity 1 will help you on your own to develop an action plan, or help a few of you to discuss and plan together. We recommend that action planning takes part in a group or team as ultimately it can only work with everyone's contributions. However, there are a few occasions when you might wish or need to do some action planning on your own. For example, you might undertake some of the individual learning activities in this resource and want to analyse the evidence you have collected to make a plan for your own development or to change the way you work with patients/residents. Here is an activity that you can try.

Individual activity

This activity is for anyone who has contributed to gathering evidence or who has done the learning activities in this resource.

You will need:

- approximately 30–45 minutes;
- your notebook with any observations, reflections, notes you have made alone or with your buddy;
- patient/ narratives or conversations if you have done any;
- your worksheet for recording learning activities with your buddy (see Chapter 1);
- any photos you have taken during your activities;
- (optional) materials, which could include felt-tip pens, paints, crayons, pastels (plus any other drawing materials you want to include);
- sticky notes.

Structured process for analysing your evidence

1. In one sitting (as a whole), read through all your notes and look at the drawings, photos etc. you have made, and form a general impression, observations, thoughts and feelings. (15 mins)
2. If an **image or metaphor has come up in your mind** whilst you were reading the evidence then draw or write it (no more than 5 mins). For example, you might have conjured up a picture or metaphor of a railway station if there is constant bustle and noise in the care setting/care home and patients/residents speak of waiting, with staff rushing about looking at their watches. This will help you get at the heart of your evidence. Alternatively, think of a **book/song/film title** or **TV programme/soap or any combination that captures what has stood out for you**. Put that on a piece of paper. (5 mins)
3. Then write the key words[1] that come immediately to your mind or imagination on sticky notes (one thing per sticky note). Do this really quickly. If you think about it too long, you may 'lose sight of the wood for the trees'. Put the sticky notes around your image/metaphor/book/song/film title or TV programme.
4. Now theme your key words, that is, put together the notes that say the same thing (perhaps in a different way) or similar things:
   a. as many themes as you like;
   b. write one theme on each sticky note and place it on your image or around your metaphor, song/film title etc.
5. Now go back to your evidence (notes, photos, worksheets etc.) to check that your themes are supported by your evidence and make any changes to your themes if necessary.
6. Reflect on your response to these themes and make notes – how they make you feel, what new thoughts you are having about them, what you are aware of now that you weren't before and how you are making sense of (interpreting) the themes and your responses to them.
7. If you have a camera, you might want to take a photo of your image etc. and themes as an aide memoir when you come to planning your learning and development.

Your themes and image/metaphor etc., responses and interpretations will help you develop your personal action plan. But first you might choose to do the *Pulling it together activity 2* below. That activity will help you to prioritise

---

[1] The key words are words that capture what stands out for you from looking at your evidence as a whole.

the themes you need to attend to in your action planning. Then there is a template for individual/informal group action planning below that you might find useful.

Small and informal group activity

This group activity would give a new facilitator a chance to practise helping people in a small group (maximum 8) to work together effectively. Whilst the topic is the same as Workshop 1 below, it is simpler and therefore more suited to a new facilitator.

If you and a small group of people who live and work in the care setting/care home have identified an area that you want to work on together, you might want to try this activity to pull together your analyses of the evidence you have gathered either individually or together, for example, with your buddy and several co-workers and patients/residents you care for.

You will need:

- approximately 1 hour;
- a group member in the role of facilitator;
- ground rules (see Chapter 2);
- themes you might have created from your own evidence (e.g. by doing the individual activity above) and which you are prepared to share with the group;
- copies of all (anonymised)[2] narrative, conversation and observation record sheets;
- a large room with chairs around the side;
- sticky notes, flipchart paper and marker pens;
- a camera.

Structured process for analysing the evidence (images and themes, narratives, conversations and observations)

1. Distribute the evidence randomly among group members and invite them to read and look at it all. Ask them to form a general impression, observations, thoughts and feelings and take notes as an aide memoir. (30 mins)
2. Invite people to write down spontaneously the key words[3] that come immediately to their minds or imaginations on sticky notes (one thing per sticky note). Encourage them to do this really quickly. Say that if they think about it too long, they might 'lose sight of the wood for the trees'.

Then you can choose between these following two options.

Option 1

3. Ask people to put the sticky notes somewhere where everyone can see them. For example, if the group is sitting in a circle of chairs put them on pieces of flipchart paper on the floor in the middle of the circle or stick the flipchart paper on the wall.
4. Ask people to theme the key words, that is, put together the sticky notes that say the same thing (perhaps in a different way) or similar things:
   a. as many themes as they like;
   b. write one theme on each sticky note and place it on your creative image;
   c. point out that this process is very similar to the theming they did in the values and beliefs clarification activity in Chapter 2 although, of course, the evidence they are working with now is different and it is being done for a different purpose.
5. Now invite people to go back to the evidence (notes, photos, worksheets etc.) to check that your themes are supported and make any changes to the themes if necessary.
6. If you have a camera, take a photo of the themes as an aide memoir for the group when they come to planning their action.

---

[2] anonymised means that the names of the person or people who have told their stories or been observed are removed or covered up and a number is allocated instead. If there are any other clues about who they are, for example, the location of their room or their title, then this should also be removed or covered up. It is important for the person responsible for storing the evidence to have a master copy of the names and the number they have been allocated, so the person can be identified if necessary, for example, to involve them in putting something right.

[3] The key words are words that capture what stands out for you from looking at your evidence as a whole.

Option 2

7. Invite people to engage in a **'speed networking'** exercise to share their impressions, feelings etc. and any pictures, colours, textures, tastes or whatever that have come to mind. They have one minute each in their pair to summarise what jumped out at them from the evidence using their picture or whatever. They do this three times, with different people. There is no discussion at this point. (6 mins)

8. Now ask people to express which of the things that people shared in the 'speed networking' rang true with their reading of the evidence. They write those things on flipchart paper. Then invite everyone to put their sticky notes next to the appropriate things on the flipchart paper.

9. Discuss whether there are some themes emerging. Are the sticky notes saying the same thing (perhaps in a different way) or similar things?
    a. Agree as many themes as they like and write the title of the theme near the cluster of sticky notes.
    b. Point out that this process is using similar principles to the theming process they did in the values and beliefs clarification activity in Chapter 2, but this time the evidence they are working with is different and it is being done for a different purpose.

10. Now invite them to go back to the evidence (notes, photos, worksheets etc.) to check that the themes are supported. People make changes to the themes if necessary.

11. If you have a camera, take a photo of the themes as an aide memoir for the group when they come to planning their action.

Both options

12. Invite group participants to reflect on their responses to these themes and make notes on:
    a. how the themes make them feel;
    b. what new thoughts they are having about the themes/what they are aware of now that they weren't before;
    c. how they are making sense of/interpreting the themes;
    d. what their responses to the themes are.

The group's themes and mind 'pictures' (if they have them), responses and interpretations will help them develop their action plan. But first the group might choose to do the *Pulling it together activity 2* a bit below. That activity will help them to identify indicators to prioritise action planning. Then there is a template for individual/informal group action planning later in this Chapter that the group might find useful.

If there is a practice development coordinating group or similar in the care setting/care home, it is really important for small informal groups to share what they are doing and their action plans with the coordinating group. This is so that the overall practice development journey will be more systematic, efficient and effective. For example, it will save time because work is not duplicated.

Pulling it together workshop 1: Analysis of evidence gathered through observations, narratives and conversations (after Boomer & McCormack, 2008; McCormack et al., 2010)

> *Workshop 1 is about helping people to analyse the evidence. The linked workshop 2 is about enabling them to compare the findings and interpretations. Both workshops can be led by an experienced facilitator. If possible, a novice facilitator could work alongside the experienced facilitator, for example making sure that pairs and small groups know what they are doing and/or are on track. The participants will be members of the practice development coordinating group or a small group of staff, patients/residents and family members who come together for this workshop.*

The purpose of Workshop 1 is the analysis of the evidence collected through observations, narratives and conversations or other similar methods.

In Chapter 5, we suggested that observations be carried out in pairs (with a buddy or colleague). We advised using the *Combined observations record sheet for feedback* to prepare your first analysis of the evidence to feed back to staff, as soon as possible after the observation.

When you get to this stage of prioritising for action planning, we suggest that all the combined observation record sheets and the patient/resident narratives and conversations record sheets are analysed further in this workshop.

The process for this analysis is experienced in a workshop format and, if the group is larger than 10, it is best run by an experienced facilitator. Groups of under 10 can be run by a care setting/care home staff member – especially someone who has gained this experience by undertaking activities in earlier chapters of this resource and in the previous activity.

You will need:

- approximately 2 hours;
- a facilitator;
- ground rules (see Chapter 2);
- copies of all (anonymised)[4] narrative, conversation and observation record sheets;
- materials, which could include felt-tip pens, paints, crayons, pastels (plus any other drawing materials you want to include); magazines and newspapers or a supply of images; scissors, glue sticks; newspaper or other floor covering if paint is being used; silver-coloured foil, coloured paper, tissue paper and card;
- a large room with chairs around the side;
- a flipchart easel, paper and marker pens;
- a camera to take pictures of the creations.

Process used for analysis of narrative, conversations and observation evidence   A structured approach to the analysis of the observation, narrative and conversation records is used. The framework progresses through seven workshop steps as follows:

1. Copies of all (anonymised) narrative, conversation and observation data are distributed randomly among group members. Ask the participants to read the evidence and form general impressions, observations, thoughts and feelings. Encourage them to make notes on these if it helps as an aide memoir to check later if they need to. Participants have 30 minutes to read the evidence.
2. When they have finished reading the evidence, ask participants to create an image of their impressions, feelings, etc. as a means of capturing the nub or the essences of the data. They can use the provided materials for

---

[4] anonymised means that the names of the person or people who have told their stories or been observed are removed or covered up and a number is allocated instead. If there are any other clues about who they are, for example, the location of their room or their title, then this should also be removed or covered up. It is important for the person responsible for storing the evidence to have a master copy of the names and the number they have been allocated, so the person can be identified if necessary, for example, to involve them in putting something right.

this creation. Participants are given 15 minutes for this activity. Remind them that they must only use the evidence that they have read and not add their own ideas. You might remember that you have had practice at ensuring that you are being true to the evidence and not adding your own thoughts when you did the values clarification activity and were theming the sticky notes.

Tell participants that if they do have an interpretation of, or very strong response to, the evidence, to make a note of it, but keep it separate ((by putting in double brackets like this, for example)). **At this stage, they may recognise something important to them, but it may not be there in the stakeholders' evidence. The participants' responses and interpretations are evidence too, so it is important that they are collected during this workshop. Their evidence will be worked with later and brought into the process of prioritising the action to be taken.**

3. Then invite each participant to join with another and take turns in 'telling the story' of their creative work and their responses or interpretations. While each person tells their story, their colleague writes down the story word for word if possible. If the colleague has a strong response to, or interpretation of what the other is saying, tell them, like above, to keep it separate ((double brackets)).

4. Using the creative image as the centre piece and the written story and other notes about the stakeholders' evidence they may have made during steps 1–3, ask each person to theme their image:
   a. as many themes as they like;
   b. write one theme on each sticky note and place it on the creative image;
   c. point out that this process is very similar to the theming they did in the values and beliefs clarification activity in Chapter 2 although, of course, the evidence they are working with now is different and it is being done for a different purpose.

5. Invite each pair to join with other pairs to form small groups to discuss the identified themes of each person. Then ask the small groups to devise 'shared themes' or categories. You must emphasise the importance of having whole-group agreement on the categories formed. Discuss also any responses and interpretations that individuals have recorded and find out whether they are shared. Record these responses and interpretations on a flipchart and indicate where they are shared and where they are individual to one person. Make sure that the flipchart is clearly marked with the title 'Responses and interpretations', the type and date of the workshop, and the facilitator's name.

6. When agreement about the categories is reached, direct each group to match their agreed categories with 'raw' evidence from the narratives, conversations and observations. Photographs are taken of the creations (to be used as a record of the analysis process and findings but also to show other stakeholders how their evidence was analysed).

7. The final sets of categories should be checked for authenticity (meaning) and resonance (ringing true) with a randomly selected sample of stakeholders who have been involved in the workshop. Once checked, the facilitator should give the final sets of categories (clearly marked with what they are, the date and name of facilitator) along with the pooled interpretations and responses of participants, to the practice development coordinating group or whoever is coordinating the evaluation and prioritisation for action planning.

8. Evaluate the workshop and encourage participants to use the worksheet to record their learning about person-centred care (see Chapter 8) that day as soon as possible whilst everyone's memory is fresh.

Pulling it together workshop 2: Comparing findings and interpretations

Workshop 2 follows on from Workshop 1 and requires an experienced facilitator working if possible with a new or less experienced facilitator as a learning opportunity for the beginner. As many participants as possible from Workshop 1 should attend, but it is good to have new participants too, as they will be more questioning and take less for granted.

The final sets of categories identified from the observations, narratives and conversations are now ready to compare with other evidence gathered using audit and evaluation tools.

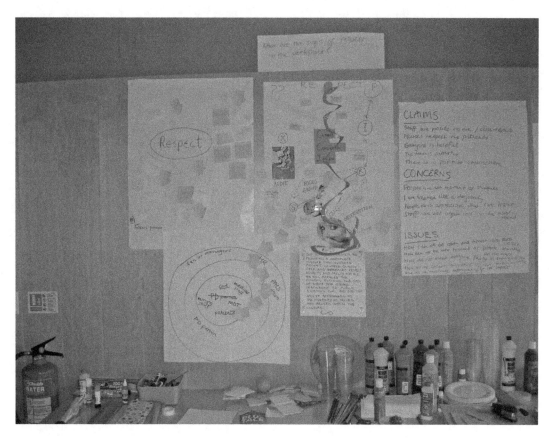

Fig. 6.3 Example of a poster made in a workshop.

The purpose of this second workshop is to compare (look for similarities and differences) between the final sets of categories identified from the observations, narratives and conversations identified in Workshop 1 and the findings that are already available in the care setting/care home. These findings might be inspection reports, quality audits previously carried out by the setting/home, the findings that were gathered by stakeholders using the Quick Evaluation (see Chapter 2 material on the companion website) to raise the profile of values and beliefs in the setting/home, the team culture tool or effective workplace culture handout (see Chapter 5). Also, don't forget the flipcharts and collages etc. that might have been produced from activities like the workshop on workplace culture (see companion website) and stakeholder meetings.

Where there are similarities, this strengthens your understanding of where the setting/home is starting off from on the practice development journey. The differences enrich the findings and give you a much more in-depth view of that starting point and particularly what the views and experiences of patients/residents are. Such a deepened understanding will enable you and your colleagues, the practice development coordinating group and other stakeholder groups to explain to themselves why they are where they are and whether the care and service given is person-centred or not.

In a cardiac care unit, many staff recognised that some aspects of care and services were not person-centred; rather, they were organised around the needs of the unit or the staff rather than the patients and families. Some staff in the unit had believed their care was already very person-centred, but as the practice development project progressed, they came to accept that it wasn't.

You will need:

- approximately 2 hours;
- a facilitator;
- copies of final sets of categories identified from the observations, narratives and conversations and the numeric findings from the audit and evaluation tools that have been used;
- photographs of the creations made in Workshop 1 above (i.e. if creations were made);
- materials, which could include highlighters, felt-tip pens, paints, crayons, pastels (plus any other drawing materials you want to include); magazines and newspapers or a supply of images; scissors, glue sticks;
- a large room with tables and chairs to accommodate small groups of six;
- a flipchart easel, paper and marker pens.

Key activities

In advance, identify/mark each category from the final sets of categories from the observations, narratives and conversations with a different colour or symbol, as shown in the margin here (shapes can be drawn with felt-tip pens).

At the workshop, if you have creations from Workshop 1, put them or photos of them up on the wall or on the tables.

1. Put a full set of findings, that is, the marked categories and the findings gained from the audit and evaluation tools, on each table. You will need a full set per six people coming to the workshop, so if there are 12 people, then you will need two full sets.
2. Invite participants to read the whole set, passing them around the table until everyone has seen them. Ask the participants to form general impressions, observations, thoughts and feelings and encourage them to make notes on these if it helps as an aide memoir to check later if they need to. (30 mins)
3. Ask them to mark similarities between the findings of the marked categories and the numeric findings with the symbol you allocated prior to the workshop.

For example, the quick evaluation tool about the care setting/care home was used to gather evidence in a learning disability unit and the observer noted that there was:

- no facility for residents to use a telephone in private;
- inconsistent encouragement for people to stay active and do things for themselves;
- poor information notices about outings or activities and often information was left up and out of date;
- no access to the kitchen for residents.

In addition, the observer recorded that there was no evidence that showed residents exercising their self-determination; rather, it was noted that a particular resident had to ask his carer for permission to phone his mother and another was not allowed to carry any money when he went out to his workplace each day.

And if categories from the observations, narratives and conversations included *choice, privacy, loss of independence, lack of self-determination*, then you would see that these evaluation data provide more evidence of your categories and you can be more certain that the evidence is strong. On the other hand, the data may show up something that didn't come out in the final set of categories and that information might be key; for example, that there is no residents committee or way that residents can have a collective voice in decision-making about their day-to-day lives and home environment. So a new theme of *decision-making* would have been identified.

4. Invite each group to make a poster showing which categories have been added to and how, and the new themes that are emerging for that group. Individual and shared responses to the evidence should be noted but kept separate. (30 mins)

5. Present the group posters to other small groups and discuss new evidence/themes that have emerged to come to an agreement that the new themes are shared and that they are firmly grounded in the data. When there is agreement, these new shared themes are called categories. Responses and interpretations are also presented and discussed for similarities and differences. Record these responses and interpretations on a flipchart and indicate where they are shared and where they are individual to one person. Make sure that the flipchart is clearly marked with the title 'Responses and interpretations', the type of workshop, date and the facilitator's name.

6. Photographs are taken of the posters (to be used as a record of the analysis process and findings and also to show other stakeholders how their evidence was analysed).

7. Now ask each group to match the new agreed categories with 'raw' evidence collected by audit and evaluation tools on their poster. Invite them to add their evidence.

8. The final sets of categories should be checked for authenticity (being genuine/real) and resonance (ringing true for everyone) with a randomly selected sample of stakeholders who have been involved in the workshop. Once checked, the facilitator should give the final sets of categories (clearly marked with what they are, the date and name of facilitator) along with the pooled interpretations and responses of participants, to the practice development coordinating group or whoever is coordinating the evaluation and prioritisation for action planning.

9. Evaluate the workshop and encourage participants to use the worksheet to record their learning about person-centred care (see Chapter 8) today as soon as possible whilst everyone's memory is fresh.

Please visit **www.wiley.com/go/practicedevelopment/workbook** to find a template (and a worked example) for recording key learning arising from these practice development workshops and evaluation activities.

Pulling it together activity 2: Individual/informal group activity for identifying indicators to prioritise action planning

In the *Pulling it together activity 1* (above), either as an individual or as part of a small, informal group, you will have established (1) your final set of themes from the evaluation evidence and (2) a collection of information about your own or the group's responses to and interpretations of that evidence. This final set and collection of information are metrics! Remember in Chapter 4 that we said that a *metric* is any set or collection of information or evidence, either quantitative or qualitative. Now you have created two metrics!

The final part of pulling it together is to establish priorities or *indicators* for action. Back in Chapter 4, we explained that an *indicator* is a particular sort of metric that indicates issues or areas that may be worth investigating.

Individual activity

To recap, the purpose of this activity is to help you to take forward the work you did in *Pulling it together activity 1*. There you developed your themes and an image/metaphor etc. to help you develop your personal action plan. This activity here will help you to prioritise the themes you need to attend to in your action planning. For example, your themes might be: *Rushing patients/residents through meals; Care organised around needs of staff; Wanting to learn, but reacting defensively to feedback*. In activity 1, you also noted down your responses to each of your themes.

For example, you might have responded to the theme *Wanting to learn, but reacting defensively to feedback* by noting that you felt very *threatened by the feedback* (response) from your buddy even though s(he) gave it in the challenging, but supportive way you had agreed in your ground rules.

You also noted that you made sense of this by recognising that *you had never received feedback before from a co-worker that was intended to help you to learn. Your normal experience was that feedback was criticism and a kind of punishment for not doing something right* (interpretation). Now you have the opportunity to sort out which of the themes (and your associated responses and interpretations) are your indicators for your further learning and action.

You will need:

- approximately 30–45 minutes;
- your themes, responses and interpretations and the picture, metaphor, book/song/film/TV programme/soap titles that captured what stood out for you when you read your evaluation evidence in *Pulling it together activity 1*;
- a copy of the form entitled *Evidence summary and action plan for aims and goals based on the person-centred practice framework* (McCormack & McCance, 2010) in this chapter.

Key activities

Have your evidence and the themes, responses and interpretations that you have distilled from the evidence to hand.

Decide which sections of the *Evidence summary and action plan for aims and goals based on the person-centred practice framework* are relevant to your themes (and responses and interpretations), and decide which ones are most important to you and which you wish to prioritise. Enter the themes and evidence summary and action plan for each box of the form that is relevant to your prioritised themes and what you want to learn and develop. You now have a draft overview of your action plan.

Think about who you could share it with to refine it and to discuss the support that you will need to carry out the action plans. You may wish at that point to fill in the more detailed action plan offered later in this chapter where you spell out the support you need.

Good luck . . .

Small informal group activity

This group activity would give a new facilitator a chance to practise helping people in a small group (maximum 8) to work together effectively. Whilst the topic is the same as Workshop 3 below, it is simpler and therefore more suited to the beginning facilitator.

To recap, the purpose of this group activity is to help the group to take forward the work they did in *Pulling it together activity 1*. There the group developed themes and perhaps mind 'pictures' as well as their responses and interpretations to help them develop their action plan. This activity here will help the group prioritise the themes they need to attend to in their action planning. For example, one of the themes might be *Noise*. The response might be *feeling remorseful that ward staff have never noticed how noisy they are as they go about their work, noisy to a level that they would never tolerate in their own homes*. Their interpretation might be that *the culture of the ward (to which they now know they contribute) has hardened their sensitivity and ability to empathise with what it must be like to be a patient in this ward.*

Explain to the group that now they have the opportunity to sort out which of the themes (and their associated responses and interpretations) are indicators for your further investigation and action.

You will need:

- approximately 1 hour;
- your themes, responses and interpretations and the mind pictures from *Pulling it together activity 1;*
- copy of the form entitled *Evidence summary and action plan for aims and goals based on the person-centred practice framework* (McCormack & McCance, 2010) (see below).

Key activities

The group has the evidence and the themes, responses and interpretations that they have distilled from the evidence to hand.

As a group, they decide which sections of the *Evidence summary and action plan for aims and goals based on the person-centred practice framework* are relevant to their themes (and responses and interpretations) and then which themes are most important for patients/residents and which they wish to prioritise. They divide into pairs or threes to work on one or two of the sheets of the form. They enter the themes and evidence summary in the relevant boxes and discuss a proposed action plan for each box. (30 mins)

Each pair or three presents the box or boxes they have filled in to the whole group for discussion and to work towards agreement. When agreement is reached, the group now has a draft overview of their action plan.

This plan is based on the evidence they have collected, analysed and interpreted and the research evidence about person-centred practice that the form is based on.

Encourage the group to think about who they could share it with to refine it and to discuss the support that they will need to carry out the action plans.

Point out to the group that after that discussion, they may wish to fill in the more detailed action plan offered later in this chapter where they can spell out the support they need.

Pulling it together workshop 3: Identifying indicators and using them to prioritise action planning

> Workshop 3 follows on from Workshop 2 and requires an experienced facilitator working if possible with a new facilitator as a learning opportunity. As many participants as possible from Workshops 1 and 2 should attend, but it is good to have new participants too as they will be more questioning and take less for granted.

The final part of pulling it together is to establish priorities or indicators for action. Back in Chapter 4, we explained that an indicator is a particular sort of metric that indicates issues or areas that may be worth investigating (a metric being any set or collection of information or evidence, either quantitative or qualitative). At the end of workshop 2, metrics were established in the form of the final set of categories from the evaluation evidence and a collection of information about the group's responses to, and interpretations of, the evidence. The purpose of this workshop 3 is to discuss whether any of these metrics are indicators that are worth further investigation or attention in the practice development plan. If the group decides to use any of the action plan templates in this workbook and companion website, then these indicators will help them to prioritise what needs to be done and in what order.

You will need:

- approximately two hours (or 2 × one hour sessions);
- copies of the final sets of categories along with the pooled interpretations and responses of participants from each of the workshops above;
- copies of the photographs of creative images and posters from the prior workshops (to show others how the evidence was analysed and interpreted);
- a facilitator;
- copies of the person-centred care template (below);
- a flipchart and pens;
- a room with tables for small groups of four to six.

Key activities

In advance of the workshop, ideally the final sets of categories, responses and interpretations are typed up and circulated to group members to consider. If this is not possible then handwritten notes will do so long as they are readable by others.

At the workshop, the photos and flipcharts that summarise the work from the two previous workshops are put on the wall.

You then invite the small groups to discuss the metrics (categories, responses and interpretations). For example, they might discuss *Patients not at the centre (category), Shocking realisation by staff that care is organised around job needs and not needs of patients* (staff's response to this category) and *Culture of task rather than people focus has been sustained by us and we are blinded to this situation* (interpretation).

The indicators would then be identified. For example, the above category, response and interpretation might be identified as one of the indicators that must have priority attention. The indicators are put up on a flipchart and presented to the other groups for discussion. Help the whole group to reach agreement on the indicators and which have priority.

Using the person-centred care template (see later in this Chapter), invite the small groups to map the agreed indicators (there is a filled in template on the companion website to help you understand what we mean), then to share their mapping with the other groups. Help the whole group reach agreement on:

- the mapping;
- how an overview plan that takes the prioritised indicators into account could be made and potentially by whom. (It is likely that several mini-projects will fall out of the overview plan and each mini-project would develop its own practice development plan with reference to the overview plan (see Chapter 7));
- agree how the findings can be fed back to stakeholders to comment on before proceeding with developing the plan. For example, an exhibition of the creative images and photos from the *Pulling it together* workshops above, alongside a concise description of the categories, responses and interpretations could be displayed in the care

setting/care home. Stakeholders could be invited to write their comments on sticky notes and leave them on the exhibition. The communication plan you made using the template offered in Chapter 4 could be helpful here to ensure that all stakeholders have an opportunity to comment on these evaluation results.

It is important that their anonymised comments are recorded and fed back to the practice development coordinating group (if there is one). Using the communication plan and a structured approach to collecting the comments will give stakeholders confidence that they are being genuinely listened to as the action plans are being developed.

- set out a series of dates for regular meetings of the practice development coordinating group to look at the overview action planning guide and template to see whether it would be helpful as a framework to receive stakeholder feedback on the findings, which will subsequently be fed into the developing action plan.
- Evaluate the workshop and encourage team members to use the worksheet to record their learning about person-centred care (see Chapter 8) today as soon as possible whilst their memory is fresh.

Structured way of ensuring two-way feedback between stakeholders and practice development coordinating group				
Stakeholder name	Comments	Date	Coordinating group response to feedback overall	Tick when told stakeholder overall comments of practice development coordinating group

Practice development coordinating group: Roles and responsibilities

In the previous workshop, we have referred again to a practice development coordinating group. Before we move on to show you how the evaluation evidence can be used for overview action planning, we pull together the roles and responsibilities of such a group. To recap, a practice development coordinating group (i.e. key stakeholders in the care setting/care home) is formed when the vision statements have been agreed by all stakeholders in the setting/home. At this point, the group may develop from the initial group that coordinated the visioning activities (Chapter 3) and/or from other key stakeholders who have been identified in the early stages. The setting up of the practice development coordinating group (including establishing ground rules or ways of working or principles of engagement – whichever term you prefer) has been described in Chapter 4, whilst Chapters 5 and 6 have pointed out the group's role (in italics below) and responsibilities (bullet points below). In summary, the roles and responsibilities are likely to be:

- *Working with stakeholders in all stages of the practice development journey:*
  - identifying stakeholders;
  - developing a communication plan (see Chapter 4);
  - communicating regularly with stakeholders about the practice development journey (see Chapter 4);
  - involving and engaging relevant stakeholders in the practice development activities below.
- *Leading the measuring and evaluation baseline evidence gathering and analysis (Chapter 5 – Gathering evidence in the workplace):*
  - coordinating the gathering and analysis of the baseline evidence with stakeholders;
  - ensuring safe storage of evidence;
  - feeding back the analysis to stakeholders;
  - coordinating the development of indicators from the evidence to prioritise action planning;
  - coordinating the mapping of the indicators on the person-centred practice template;
  - feeding back the mapping to stakeholders.
- *Developing, implementing and evaluating the integrated practice development plan (Chapters 6 and 7):*
  - feeding back drafts of the plan to stakeholders for comment and suggested amendments;
  - finalising the plan and sharing with stakeholders in diverse ways (e.g. posters, newsletters);
  - inviting and receiving ideas for mini-projects from stakeholders in the setting/home and determining which ideas are most likely to progress the action plans and lead to the vision becoming reality;
  - inviting initiators and relevant stakeholders to become members of the mini-project group. Recommending the size of the group (the size will depend on the project and the size of the setting/home, but no more than eight is probably best for efficient working. Very small projects may only have two or three project members);
  - supporting the project group in implementing and evaluating the mini-projects' plans and sharing the findings of their project work;
  - giving and receiving feedback to and from mini-project groups about the project group's experiences, progress and ways of working;
  - receiving evaluation reports at agreed intervals from the mini-project groups. Using them to map progress (e.g. using the person-centred practice template and/or key milestones and target dates' pages in the overall action plan);
  - preparing overall evaluation reports of the whole practice development journey (including summaries of the mini-projects' processes and outcomes for patients/residents and staff) for the Executive team at agreed intervals.
- *Leading the development, implementation and evaluation of support systems staff and patients/residents (see Chapter 8)*
  - creating a person-centred learning environment, e.g.:
    - supporting the leader and managers in setting the strategic direction for learning in the team or in the setting/home;
    - setting up interactive noticeboards for learning activities for patients/residents and staff;
    - encouraging short reflective spaces in the working day;
    - constructively giving and receiving feedback to and from team members and patients/residents.
  - providing systems of support for work-based learning, e.g. inductive programmes, mentoring, active learning, action learning, supporting development of learning buddies;
  - modelling active learning, self-evaluation of learning and the use of enabling questions.

Person-centred practice templates

Please now visit www.wiley.com/go/practicedevelopment/workbook for a series of templates for you to use in recording the key findings from your evaluation activities and developing these into an action plan for further developing person-centred practice. Also available are some examples of these templates filled in to give you an idea how to use them. These templates and the ones below are primarily for care setting/care home team members who have professional or vocational qualifications. It is likely to be useful to a practice development coordinating group or those leading, coordinating and facilitating the development of practice in the setting/home.

> Remember to share successes and progress as time goes by.
>
> Give praise and recognition where it is due.

In Chapter 1, we presented the person-centred practice framework (McCormack & McCance, 2010) – see Figure 1.3. This framework suggests that if care teams and organisations systematically attend to the care environment and the attributes of the caregivers, this helps the caregivers to work with people in authentic ways. A philosophy of person-centred care can gradually be made real and person-centred care outcomes achieved. When used with a practice development approach, this framework provides a method for effective change in the culture and context of the setting/home. The templates further on and on the companion website build on the person-centred practice framework and will help you to bring together your key findings (from the various sources) to inform your action plans to develop person-centred care. If you already have a model for your care you may like to look at how you can use the concepts or headings within the model as a similar template.

Evidence summary and action plan for aims and goals based on the person-centred practice framework (McCormack & McCance, 2010)

Attributes or prerequisites of the individual member of the care setting/care home team

Competent in doing the job	Effective interpersonal skills	Commitment to the job	Clarity of beliefs and values	Knowing 'self'
Evidence Summary				
Action Plan				

The context in which care is delivered – the care environment

Appropriate skill mix	Systems that help shared decision-making	Effective staff relationships	Supportive organisational systems	Sharing of power	Potential for innovation and risk taking	Physical environment
Evidence Summary						
Action Plan						

Delivery of care through a range of activities – Care processes				
Working With Patient/ Resident's Beliefs And Values	Engagement	Sympathetic Presence	Sharing Decision- Making	Providing For Holistic Care
Evidence Summary				
Action Plan				

Results of effective person-centred care – Person-centred outcomes

Satisfaction with care	Involvement with care	Feeling of well-being	Creating a therapeutic culture
Evidence Summary			
Action Plan			

Overview action planning guide

This guide and the overview action planning template in the companion website can be used by the practice development coordinating group. It can be used by an individual who is leading, evaluating and facilitating change in the care setting/care home, an informal or a formal group (e.g. mini-project group) or it can be used as the basis for more detailed planning for mini-projects.

Overview action planning is long-term planning of action and development designed to achieve a particular endpoint (aim or goal) or set of end-points (aims or goals). It is built on the premise of achieving success. It is thus concerned with deciding where the setting/home wants to be and how it is going to get there in broad terms. It should reflect the setting/home's values and vision. The plan will often set out what are called aims or goals, objectives and key milestones, and targets for the duration of the strategy. Aims are the overall statements of where the organisation is going. Objectives detail how the endpoint (aim or goal) will be achieved. Milestones are a way in which the objective to be reached is broken down into achievable short-term targets. These targets make clear what needs to be achieved by a certain point in time. Targets can be used as criteria to evaluate progress towards an objective.

The wording for the practice development aims and objectives can be taken from the setting/home vision statement that has already been developed by stakeholders. The initial evaluation evidence that may have been collated in the Evidence summary and action planning template above or the Person-centred care templates on the companion website can be used to stimulate further discussion about the actions that need to be taken to achieve the endpoints. These actions are also likely to include how work-based, active learning (see Chapter 8) systems and processes for developing staff can be built into the working day.

Now go to **www.wiley.com/go/practicedevelopment/workbook** where you will find an overview action planning template that can be downloaded and copied for your use. Before you decide to use the overview action planning template, we advise you to check with your manager whether there is a required action planning format for your organisation. If there is, you could assess whether you could work in the ideas presented here within your required format.

SMART and SMARTER goals

Using this device can help you develop achievable goals. It can be used by anyone developing an action plan whether it is for individual learning or for the overview or mini-project action plans. So the device can be used by anyone in the setting/home as well as the practice development coordinating group, an individual who is leading, evaluating and facilitating change and an informal or a formal group (e.g. mini-project group).

SMART goals
Specific • Well-defined • Clear to anyone who has an elementary knowledge of the project
Measurable • Know if the goal is obtainable and how far away completion is • Know when it has been achieved
Agreed upon • Agreement with all stakeholders or participants on what the goal should be
Realistic • Can be achieved within the availability of resources including knowledge, skill and time
Time-based • Enough time to achieve the goal • Is not time-expensive in a way that would affect project performance

Energising • Produces positive effects and motivates further action
Recorded • Documented and shared with all stakeholders or participants

Note: **E** can also stand for excitement and **R** for risk

Chapter 7 Mini-projects: Ongoing and Integrated Action, Evaluation, Learning and Planning

Contents

Introduction

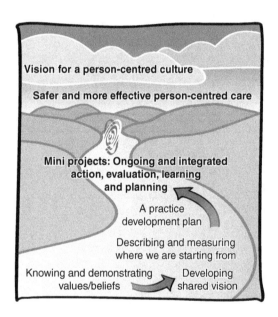

Fig. 7.1 The next step: Mini-projects and ongoing, integrated action, evaluation, learning and planning.

The examples of mini-projects in this chapter are relevant for everyone working in the care setting. The examples describe real projects carried out by teams and patients/residents. Examples range from creating better hospital day rooms, a more homely environment, making mealtimes a social occasion, to offering meaningful activities. The examples will give you a sense of what is possible and achievable.

The whole chapter is relevant for you when you get involved in a mini-project, as a project member or small group member that is focusing on a specific thing in the project. The chapter will give you ideas on how to set up the project and small groups, lead them and develop action plans together. Some of the resources in here might be of interest to students and other learners.

Practice Development Workbook for Nursing, Health and Social Care Teams, First Edition. Jan Dewing, Brendan McCormack, and Angie Titchen.
© 2014 John Wiley & Sons, Ltd. Published 2014 by John Wiley & Sons, Ltd.
Companion website: www.wiley.com/go/practicedevelopment/workbook

Now you have got together your practice development plan you might feel that you are about to set off on your practice development journey. Well, if you have been doing the activities and workshops as set out in this resource, your journey to a person-centred care has, in fact, already begun.

Your practice development plan might have identified a number of mini-projects that individuals or more usually small groups of team members patients/residents/families can do together. As starting small is a good, feasible way to get going on the overall plan, Chapter 6 offers you help on getting the structure and processes for mini-projects in place. Now, this won't be entirely new to you if you have been involved in the activities in this resource because the ways mini-projects are set up are based on person-centred values. This means that the structure and processes are going to be the same or similar to those underpinning the practice development coordinating group (if you have one set up) or small group work in the activities in previous chapters. If you liken this similarity to Figure 7.2, each of the parts/florets (mini-project structure) of the broccoli echoes the structure of the whole broccoli (practice development coordination structure in the care setting/home). The same similarity recurs when sub-groups or stakeholder relationships are set up in the florets (mini-projects). Look closely and you will see that each floret has a structure of miniature florets that again mirror the whole vegetable. In other words, each part contributes the whole in a consistent and coherent way. The values integrate all the structures and processes of any number of mini-projects. Together they turn the vision into reality. Structures and processes that mirror person-centredness are vital in helping create a person-centred culture in your setting.

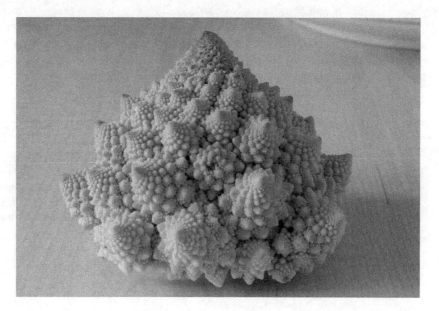

Fig. 7.2 The parts mirror the whole structure.
(Source: Wikimedia commons)

Think back to the person-centred practice framework (see Chapter 1) and the need to consider the *care environment* in the development of a person-centred culture. Do you remember that the second circle from the outside in Figure 1.3 represents the *care environment*? This environment is your care setting. It includes:

- the development of effective staff relationships and power sharing as a team and with patients/residents and families;
- organisational systems that are supportive;
- the potential for innovation and risk taking.

The setting up of mini-projects and their systems of support is an excellent way of developing your workplace. What happens is that as a person-centred way of working becomes established in the mini-projects, this way of working can start to filter into the way the setting/home is run and goes about its everyday care business. It is as if the mini-projects are small laboratories for experimenting with new ways of working, learning and being. These new ways then spill over into everyday working with the team, patients/residents and families. Mini-projects offer the team freedom to work autonomously (but to an overall plan), and to be innovative and take assessed risks. The point of doing this is that it contributes to better experiences with care and can enhance the well-being of patients/residents and team members.

Before getting to the point of setting up mini-projects, the following phases (or something similar to these) will have taken place:

1. Working out the shared values and beliefs and vision for the stakeholders and service/home.
2. Converting the key purposes into vision statements.
3. Using the vision statements to identify core evaluation questions and stakeholder Claims, Concerns and Issues to identify sub-questions.
4. Identifying what evidence is already available that applies locally and is retrievable within the care setting/care home.
5. Identifying what evidence is not available or retrievable within the care setting/care home and how you will gather it.
6. Collating available evidence and gathering new evidence.
7. Prioritising to form a practice development plan.
8. Knowing what other plans exist in your care setting/care home and/or organisation to link work up together.
9. Creating an integrated evaluation, action and learning plan, i.e. a practice development plan.

A final word about mini-projects undertaken by individuals: these are likely to focus on an individual's learning about how to work in person-centred ways. Therefore, the materials in Chapter 8 Learning in the workplace might be more useful for some individuals than some of those in this chapter. Having said that, the examples of the mini-projects provided here may provide inspiration or some guidance for work in your care setting. The examples you will read about in here are not perfect by any means – because developing practice isn't! Do not feel you need to copy or replicate them – use them to stimulate ideas about what your service/home needs at this time. Follow the principles but do it in the way that suits the people living there.

Resources in this chapter

- **Examples of mini-projects** – to inspire you and show what is possible, we include excerpts from:
  - an article by Helen Hunnisett, a physiotherapist who came to see the value of staff from different professions and other stakeholders coming together to work on small projects and working groups;
  - an example of a mini-project about workplace culture observations by Jan Dewing and colleagues;
  - the final report of the Older Persons National Practice Development Programme in the Republic of Ireland (2007–2009) (McCormack et al., 2010). This example is the result of two years of development in some homes. They could give you lots of ideas for beginning mini-projects with your colleagues and residents. Moreover, a new guide (Health Service Executive, 2010) from this programme is now available and could be used in addition to this chapter.

These projects are focused on older people's services and may therefore not seem directly relevant to people working in other services. However, it can still be useful to look at the processes used within the projects and see what learning can be taken from them.

- **A guide to mini-project structure and processes** – this guide shows you the structure, i.e. roles, responsibilities, work organisation and ways of working and processes like action planning.
- **Leading a project/working/action group** – this resource poses a number of questions to help you prepare yourself if you have volunteered or been invited to lead a group connected to a mini-project. The questions could help you to reflect upon what you know and don't know and to develop a learning plan.
- **Mini-project action planning template** – a blank template is offered for you to use. A filled in one shows how you can use it to develop a project action plan.

In Chapter 9, there are Frequently Asked Questions that are relevant *to mini-projects*.

Examples of mini-projects

The following extracts and examples are useful to give you ideas of what is possible. The mini-projects are based on the same practice development principles, structures and processes as those presented in this resource.

1. 'Light bulb moment'

The first example is an excerpt from an article written by Helen Hunnisett, a physiotherapist. Her work was published in the *International Practice Development Journal*, a free online journal that we featured in Chapter 1 of this resource. You can access the journal by following the simple instructions on the home page of the Foundation of Nursing Studies website (www.fons.org).

As a member of a busy team in health care, as in most units or wards, it is too easy to just 'do your job' and not to see the issues that patients, relatives and visitors see. The staff-centred and task culture for us was long standing and unchallenged. I recall when I went to work there I initially felt very uneasy about some of the practices I saw, but I soon felt powerless to challenge the culture and our physiotherapy team subconsciously disassociated itself from the ward area, including the nurses. We assessed, we treated but rarely became involved in discharge planning and stood back while the nursing and occupational therapy teams facilitated the discharge of patients. However, the length of stay for patients was immense. Over time the number of patients who had been in the unit for over six months began to increase. The whole service was fragmenting and strong characters amongst the ward team appeared to rule the unit and I learned never to challenge them. I think I didn't really know how to do that.

The road to change started on a staff away day in 2008 where all staff were invited to express their feelings, positive and negative and questions they had about the unit. This was what I called my 'light bulb' moment (Mezirow, 1990, p14). The majority of staff, who to be honest, I had probably never really spoken to, were stating exactly the same views as me. We could all see that we wanted to be proud of our unit and do the best for each individual that comes through our doors. Yet we could all see that we were miles away from that and could even identify how it could be better. At the same event, we were facilitated to work together to create our own vision (Warfield and Manley, 1990; Manley, 1992). The vision statement created by us gave us, I felt, a sense of the autonomy to challenge and also support anyone who was not upholding the standards that we all set.

After this other practice development activities started to be introduced such as working or project groups and clinical supervision. The working groups were organised around topics that had been identified by us, the team, as areas for improvement and involved multiple disciplines of varying grades working collaboratively to identify what we did well, causes of ineffective working or gaps in our practice. In the past any changes seemed to come about simply by two pathways, that of a manager telling you it was to happen or a couple of staff members coming up with an idea and hoping it would be carried out by all staff; neither of which seemed to have any impact or be sustained. However, this new method saw staff raising questions, making observations and feeding back the information to their colleagues. Very slowly the culture started to change . . .

Hunnisett (2011) © *International Practice Development Journal* and reproduced by their kind permission.

2. Inconsistency and contradictions

The second example is the abstract of the article written by Jan Dewing and her colleagues. This article is also published in the *International Practice Development Journal*. Just click on the link and register for free.

Aims and objectives: The overall aim of this mini project was to collaboratively engage in a learning activity that would provide evidence about the workplace culture to be used to inform other aspects of practice development work. The objectives were: to enhance observation skills; contribute to a team development activity; share and develop critical questions for use with local practice development action planning and build up active commitment to practice development work within the group.

Design: A small pilot project embedded within a larger complex emancipatory practice development programme.

Method: An unstructured observation method was used and followed up with facilitated critical reflection and dialogue.

Results: The overall theme was Inconsistency and Contradictions. Seven contradictory sub-themes were found: light and dark; cleanliness and clutter; quiet and noise; calmness and busyness; conversation and chatter; communal and bedside; respect and disrespect.

Conclusions: This pilot project shows that multi-dimensional small scale outcomes can be identified very early on in practice development. Testing and developing a practice development method and processes for wider scale use in an organisation is an important feature of micro level practice development within health-care organisations.

Implications for practice: A group of practitioners can learn to carry out and collate findings from observations within their own workplace. Becoming critically aware of context and culture is a process and it needs to be facilitated to ensure that learning progresses to collaborative action. Outcomes can be maximised by building in facilitation to promote reflection and dialogue. An observation method on workplace culture can form part of a diagnostic and evaluation portfolio at practice level which can contribute to larger scale evaluation, quality and clinical governance agendas.

Dewing et al. (2011) © *International Practice Development Journal* and reproduced by their kind permission.
(www.fons.org/library/journal/volume1-issue1/article3)

3. Older Persons National Practice Development Programme in the Republic of Ireland (2007–2009) (McCormack et al., 2010)

Hundreds of residential care staff and older people collaborated and participated in this programme. Eighteen care facilities for older people were included.

- The final report of the Older Persons National Practice Development Programme in the Republic of Ireland (2007–2009) (McCormack et al., 2010) is well worth downloading from: www.lenus.ie/hse/
- Enhancing Care for Older People: A Guide to Practice Development Processes to Support and Enhance Care in Residential Settings for Older People, June 2010: www.hse.ie/eng/services/Publications/corporate/NursingMidwifery%20Services/Enhancing%20Care%20for%20Older%20People.pdf
- Or a short summary can be found at: www.britishgerontology.org/DB/gr-editions-2/generations-review/the-implementation-of-a-model-of-person-centred-pr.html
- The outcomes of the programme for older people and the teams make inspirational reading. The report presents the evaluation evidence from which a huge variety of projects were grown.
- Developed from the Irish programme, a new guide to practice development processes to support and enhance care in residential settings for older people has been published by the Health Service Executive (2010). We recommend it as a further resource for your work and your workplace.

 For details please see the companion web site at **www.wiley.com/go/practicedevelopment/workbook**.

Mini-projects: Guide to structure and processes

> This guide is to help those who have been asked or have volunteered to set up a mini-project

Usually a mini-project emerges from the overall practice development plan, which in turn evolves from team members, patients/residents and families collecting their baseline evaluation evidence in a variety of ways. The initial idea for the mini-project can be presented to the practice development coordinating group (or something similar) by any stakeholder in the service/home. It may have been decided that it is the role and responsibility of the practice development coordinating group to give mini-projects the go-ahead, monitor their progress and contribution to the practice development journey and provide necessary support (see Chapter 5 for suggested roles and responsibilities of a practice development coordinating group).

Mini-project group structure

Structure here refers to the roles, responsibilities, organisation of work and ways of working of all those in a mini-project group.

Mini-projects: Roles and responsibilities

The roles and responsibilities of a mini-project group are to plan, implement and evaluate the project work with stakeholders and to report back to an overall coordinating group (if there is one) at agreed intervals. They are also to be enthusiastic and hopeful about making a positive difference when talking about the work with others. The mini-group's roles and responsibilities are similar, smaller versions with a smaller scale, if you like, of those of the practice development coordinating group (see Chapter 6). So your roles (in italics below) and responsibilities (bullet points) might look like this (**don't panic, if you have done any of the activities in earlier chapters of this resource, you will already have had experience of some of these things, and those of you haven't, you will find some of the skills transferable**):

- *Working with stakeholders in your project:*
  - familiarising yourself with the overall practice development plan;
  - identifying the relevant stakeholders;
  - developing a communication plan with those stakeholders (see Chapter 4);
  - communicating regularly with stakeholders about the practice development journey (see Chapter 4);
  - involving and engaging relevant stakeholders in the practice development activities below.
- *Leading the measuring and evaluation baseline evidence gathering and analysis for the project:*
  - refamiliarising yourself with the vision for person-centred care that all stakeholders, including yourself, had the opportunity to contribute to, and discussing how your mini-project is going to help achieve that vision;
  - identifying which evaluation questions in the overall practice development plan are relevant to your project;
  - through carrying out a Claims, Concerns and Issues activity with your stakeholders, establish whether you need to identify further evaluation questions from the issues that are particularly relevant to your project (see Chapter 4);
  - deciding whether the baseline evidence that is already available in the home is sufficient for your needs, whether you need some supplementary evidence and if yes, how you would collect and analyse it (Chapter 4);
  - ensuring safe storage of extra evidence gathered – if the practice development coordinating group has decided to keep all the evidence in the home together to ensure confidentiality, then you will need to make sure it is given to the right person;
  - gathering and analysing any extra evidence (Chapter 5);
  - feeding back this analysis to stakeholders to check whether it rings true;
  - identifying indicators from the project evidence to prioritise action planning for the project;
  - coordinating the mapping of the indicators on the person-centred practice template (see companion website);
  - creating an action or practice development plan for the project (there is a template further on);
  - feeding back the plan to stakeholders for comment and suggestions.

> ### Developing, implementing and evaluating the mini-project plan
>
> Going on a practice development journey and carrying out a mini-project plan of integrated evaluation – learning – action is more like journeying along a spiral than going in a straight line. This is because the same things, such as using person-centred language and avoiding stereotyping or labelling people, creating meaningful activities, creating a learning environment and developing a person-centred culture are revisited again and again. This is to see whether the action or the learning has been put into practice and whether it has been effective.

- *Developing, implementing and evaluating the mini-project plan:*
  - feeding back drafts of the plan to stakeholders for comment and suggested amendments;
  - finalising the plan and sharing with stakeholders in diverse ways (e.g. posters, newsletters);
  - carrying out the development work and gathering evidence to find out whether your intended actions are successful or not and why;
  - discussing the evidence to see whether you need to change tack, revise your plans, i.e. using this ongoing evidence to inform your revised aims, plans and actions or whether to continue going as before
  - preparing and submitting short evaluation reports at agreed intervals to the practice development coordination group
  - using these reports to map progress (e.g. using the person-centred practice template and/or key milestones and target dates pages in the action plan)
- *Making use of support systems for team members and older people*
  - engage in systems of support provided by the organisation, home or practice development coordinating group, e.g. mentorship, coaching, learning supervision, active learning, action learning, supporting development of learning buddies;
  - use these forms of support to reflect on your own, and to facilitate others', learning and development; review and evaluate your own and others' performance of your roles in the mini-project;
  - develop your facilitation of learning and practice development skills;
  - negotiate short reflection and evaluation spaces in your mini-project group meetings for learning from your shared experiences and group working.

Mini-projects: Work organisation / ways of working

Once the mini-project group members have been identified and invited to join the project (this may have been done by the practice development coordinating group or by the initiator of the idea), it is important to ensure efficiency, effectiveness and success of the project. This is done by discussing and negotiating the structure of the group in terms of how you are going to organise the work itself and how you will work together. You will also need to decide group member roles. For example, one group member might be the group lead/facilitator, and another may be responsible for stakeholder collaboration inclusion and participation in the project.

Things to think about when inviting people to join the mini-project group

- Who are the key stakeholders that are relevant to the project and are enthusiastic about developing person-centred care?
- Who has the skills, capacity and potential willingness to join the project group?
- How can we ensure that the project group membership reflects the spread of relevant key stakeholders?
- How big a group do we need?
- How often will the group need to meet, where and at what time?
- Who will take the group lead/facilitation/coordination role?
- How will the work of the group be resourced?

Once the group is established, group members will need to:

- discuss and agree the remit of the group;
- clarify their roles within the group (see Chapter 3) and negotiate these roles with other group members;
- establish ground rules or person-centred ways of working together (see Chapter 2 for a handout);
- agree how meetings will be run, whether the templates for efficient agenda setting and note-taking, presented in Chapter 2, could be modified for this project;

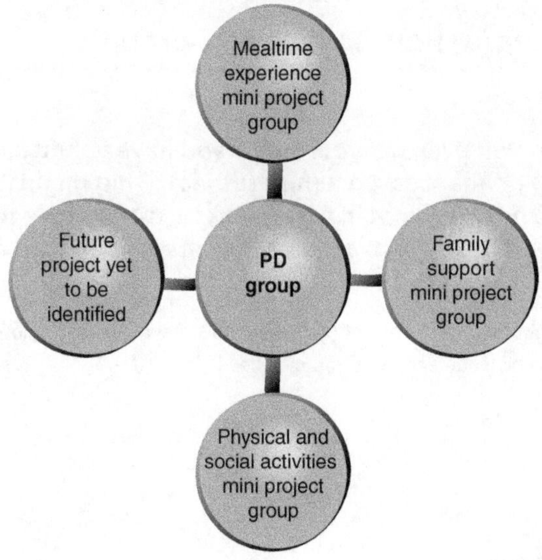

Fig. 7.3 The structure at Sunnyside Care Home, South of England.

- they may also wish to review the questions (and action points) generated by stakeholders at the workshop on Current evaluation methods within your organisation (see Chapter 4) to get a sense of where stakeholders are starting from in terms of the practice development journey.

Another way of showing the relationship between the main group and the mini-project groups is from Sunnyside Care Home in the South of England (see Figure 7.3), but equally any kind of mini-project in any kind of service or setting could be placed in the outer circles.

Mini-project processes

Just as mini-project structure is informed by person-centred values and practice development principles, the same goes for the processes that the mini-project group members use in their work together and with all stakeholders.

Group processes Project group sessions are based on the practice development principles of collaboration, inclusion and participation, so processes need to be democratic and facilitative. For example, the Claims, Concerns and Issues process can be used to set the content of the sessions and will ensure that everyone at the meeting has their say. Facilitating such sessions and helping people to be reflective requires certain skills. It may be that you need to develop such skills. Chapter 8 contains resources to help you to do so and thereby to work effectively with groups and create a group culture of effectiveness/learning. Examples of resources there include how to do a process review of your sessions in order to evaluate, for example, whether you are using person-centred language and whether you are really being collaborative, inclusive and participative with people in the group.

Action planning In previous chapters and on the companion website, a number of resources on action planning are offered, such as activities to identify indicators to prioritise action planning, using a stakeholder communication plan, the planning roles and responsibilities of a practice development coordinating group, person-centred practice templates and an overview action planning template. These are all relevant to planning mini-projects. To show you how, we have modified below the overview practice development plan template (see companion website) for an imaginary mini-project. But don't forget to check with your manager whether there is a required format for action planning in your setting/home. Before you look at our plan for the imaginary mini-project, have a look at the following template we have created to help you prepare for leading a working/action/project group.

Sheet 7.1: Leading a project/working/action or learning group

This template will help you prepare yourself if you have volunteered or been invited to lead a group connected to a mini-project. This might be the project group that is leading and coordinating the work or it may be a working/action group that is set up by the project group to do specific pieces of work.

The questions that follow next might help you to reflect upon what you know and don't know and to develop a learning plan to help you develop the knowledge and skills you may need.

What do I know about:
- setting up a group;
- teamwork;
- group processes;
- leading/facilitating a group/team;
- how to offer high challenge/high support to group/team members to help them learn through working on the project;
- helping people to reflect about themselves as a person and worker interacting with others in the care setting and to solve problems effectively;
- helping create a person-centred group/team culture in their work together;
- facilitating an action plan that is owned by all group/team members?

Where are the gaps in my knowledge?

What experience do I have that I can draw on to help me lead a group?

How can others in the group help me and what skills and strengths do they have to offer the group and our work?

How aware am I of how effective I am in leading a group?

How do I evaluate my own and others' effectiveness in leading/contributing to the effective working of the group/team?

What are my strengths, weaknesses, opportunities and threats?

What do I need to learn?

What resources do I need?

Who can help me learn/assess the resources?

Would any of the resources in Chapter 8 be helpful to me?

Sheet 7.2: Mini-project action planning template

(adapted from International Practice Development Collaborative template (Dewing & Titchen, 2007)

Practice development aims[1] to which this mini-project relates:

Mini-project practice development aims[2]:

Mini-project practice development statements of intent or objectives[3]:

Practice development aims:

Practice development statements of intent or objectives:

Title of project/ Practice development work:

Action plan   Date: _____

Objective: What do I/we need to achieve? (your indicators will guide you here)

Timescale: When do I/we need to have achieved the practice development objective?

Insert date: _____

---

[1] This is a general or overarching aim that will be documented in the overview action plan in your care setting/home (Chapter 6 (see companion website)). It is helpful to think of aims as nouns, i.e. something that you are aiming to get to.
[2] These are more specific smaller aims that are linked to the overarching aim.
[3] The statements of intent or objectives set out how the project will achieve the aims. It is helpful to think of these as verbs because they involve taking action.

Resources: What resources do I/we need to have available to achieve my/our objective? (Consider any resources that are already available to you.)

Support/challenge available: What support and challenge do I/we need to achieve my/our objective?

Support:

Challenge:

Desired outcomes for workplace culture (see person-centred template)

Patients/residents/family/visitor outcomes:

Team members/volunteer/team outcomes:

Care setting/home outcomes:

Forcefield analysis: What factors may help or hinder the achievement of my/our objectives? Do the following for each objective.

1. Group members identify factors that may help them to achieve their objective (driving forces).
2. Group members identify factors that may hinder them in achieving their objective (restraining forces).
3. Each member considers each force and gives it a value (for example, 0 = not relevant/no force, 1 = low force, 2 = medium force, 3 = high force).
4. Add up the score for each factor.
5. Factors with the most points need to receive the most attention.
6. Plan how to overcome the restraining forces and harness the driving forces to achieve the objective.

Driving forces	Restraining forces

If you haven't already done the Strengths, Weaknesses, Opportunities and Threats (SWOT) activity in Chapter 5, now might be a good time to do it.

Chart: What activities do I/we need to undertake to achieve my/our objective? (Note: one chart for each objective)

Key activity	Timescale for activity (start/end dates)	Lead and key stakeholders, participants	Stakeholders I/we will account to about my/our work

What evidence will I/we need to have to evaluate the achievement of the objectives? (Refer back to desired outcomes with workplace culture.)

What methods and criteria for success will I/we use to evaluate the achievement of the key activities and objectives? Who will help to check that the evidence does show that achievement?

Who needs to know about the action plan (e.g. stakeholders, managers)?

How will I/we evaluate our learning about practice development and workplace culture?

Date action plan agreed
Insert date: _____

PRACTICE DEVELOPMENT participants' names: (all group to sign)

_____

_____

_____

_____

Year 1

Activity/milestone	Lead	Target date	Comments about achievement and progress

Sheet 7.3: Example: Filled in mini-project action planning template

(adapted from International Practice Development Collaborative template, Dewing & Titchen, 2007)

Here is an example of the action planning template filled in for a mini-project involving a multi-professional health-care surgical team. The topic is helping patients post-operatively to manage and begin to adjust to having a new, probably permanent colostomy. A group of surgical ward staff (registered nurses and a health-care assistant), a clinical nurse specialist in stoma care and a surgical registrar have gathered data to evaluate the service they offer such patients. One of the approaches they used was patient stories that were collected when patients from their ward attended an out-patient clinic 3 months after discharge. The team has now reflected upon their analysis of the stories and agreed that they all fall short, in various ways, of providing a service that helps patients to engage in self-care of their stomas and to begin to accept the stoma as part of themselves as a person.

At the same time that the stories were gathered, observations of care were carried out by two ward nurses, which revealed that the ward nurses rely on the stoma nurse to teach patients how to self-care and that they (and the ward leader) see their role as merely changing the bag when necessary. When the observations were fed back to them, the nurses were prepared to admit that they disliked this work and (as shown in the patient stories), they tended to avoid it, which sometimes resulted in stoma bags leaking. The patient stories revealed how distressing many patients had found soiling the bed or chair. A few patients recalled barely disguised disgust on the faces of one or two nurses and the off-hand manner of the medical surgical team when they asked questions about their stoma care and how they would cope at home, as they either lived alone or definitely did not want their spouse or partner to do this for them. Another frequent question that the patients said they wanted, but didn't feel comfortable, to ask: what did this surgery mean for their sex lives? How could they ever consider having sexual relations again and how could they cope with the impact this would have on their spouse/partner?

What has surprised the team now is that the vision that everyone in the surgical unit created together for person-centred patient care in the unit is so very different from the stark reality of the patients' stories and the observations of care in this ward. So they want to do something about it. Therefore, they have offered this mini-project topic to the practice development coordinating group in the unit and have been given the go-ahead. They have used the findings of the baseline evaluation and the overall unit practice development plan to develop this (imaginary) mini-project plan for learning-acting-evaluating.

Practice development aims to which this mini-project relates:

1. *The provision of person-centred care of all patients who undergo surgery in the unit and their families*
2. *Working in genuine partnerships with patients and families*
3. *Human flourishing for patients, families and staff*

Mini-project practice development aims:

1. *The ward leader supports the nurses in extending their role to include helping patients to care for their own stomas*
2. *The clinical nurse specialist develops facilitation skills so that she can help the nursing team develop the necessary skills for supporting patients' self-care of their stoma.*
3. *Patients are supported by the ward nursing team in achieving self-care of their stoma and in accepting it and the appliance as a part of their own body and self, rather than experiencing it as a distasteful 'foreign body'.*
4. *The multi-professional team creates the conditions for patients to voice their concerns and questions, openly and without fear, during their everyday contact with patients and their spouses and partners.*

Mini-project practice development statements of intent or objectives:

1. *To develop active learning opportunities in the working day that will offer all members of the multi-professional team who work in the ward high challenge and high support.*
2. *To identify how we can all help patients and their families within our everyday work and not see it as 'yet another task to do'.*

3. *To increase our awareness of and skill in:*
   - *being really present in a sympathetic way (especially when we are busy), listening actively and asking enabling questions that create the conditions for patients and their families to talk about the stoma;*
   - *(ward nursing team) dealing with any negative feelings we may experience when helping patients to care for their stoma;*
   - *(everyone) helping them to take responsibility for self-care of their stoma and acquire knowledge and skills for doing so.*

4. *To create a person-centred workplace culture in the ward where learning, improving and evaluating practice is the way we do things around here.*

Title of mini-project *'How can we help you with your stoma?'*
Action plan   **Date:** *1 October*
Objective: What do I/we need to achieve? (your indicators will guide you here)

> *We need to:*
> - *invite the ward leader, a consultant surgeon and the patients who told their stories to become part of our mini-project team;*
> - *inform the Executive team of the hospital that we are planning this project;*
> - *help ourselves and all staff who work on the ward not to pass judgement on or blame ourselves or others for the experience of past patients but rather to focus our energy on how we can improve things together with patients for present and future care;*
> - *create active learning opportunities in our everyday work;*
> - *ward leader and nursing team leaders invited to work alongside the stoma care nurse to learn how to facilitate patients' self-care and create the conditions for helping patients to own, and adjust to, their stomas;*
> - *patients are made aware that the nurses (starting with the leaders) are learning how to help patients to care for their own stomas. They are asked for feedback on their experience of being helped, so that the leaders can learn whether their actions have been effective;*
> - *when the team leaders are working effectively, members of their team, in turn, work alongside them in the same way (i.e. they become role models);*
> - *the ward leader and consultant surgeon support this way of learning-working-evaluating in the ward and role-model it to the multi-disciplinary team on ward rounds;*
> - *everyone (including medical staff) capitalises on the buddy system the unit practice development group has set up by getting buddies ourselves and encouraging others to do so as well;*
> - *work with buddies to learn how to challenge each other sensitively and supportively about how we enable patients' self-care and acceptance of their stoma as part of themselves in a way that both learn from the challenge;*
> - *get feedback from key stakeholders about the impact of the mini-project on the care of patients with a stoma;*
> - *Recognise and praise examples of person-centred partnerships with patients and with colleagues.*

Timescale: When do I/we need to have achieved the mini-project objectives?

> *Insert date: 1 October 20—*
> *We are aware that creating a person-centred culture on the ward will be ongoing work, but within 3 months we expect to see some patients managing their own stomas and referring to their stomas as part of themselves and not a distasteful, foreign body. We expect to see the majority of patients doing this within 6 months.*

Resources: What resources do I/we need to have available to achieve my/our objective? (Consider any resources that are already available to you.)

1. *Support by the key stakeholders for this project.*
2. *Patients, past and present, on the ward.*
3. *The baseline evaluation evidence from the patient stories and observations of care.*
4. *The buddy system, supported by a training session for buddies.*
5. *Allocation of 1.5 hours every 6–8 weeks for a project group session to evaluate progress, learn from the evaluation data and change or refine this plan.*

Support/challenge available: What support and challenge do I/we need to achieve my/our objective?

Support:
1. *We can support each other in our sessions and in learning and working together on the ward and during ward rounds.*
2. *Being more aware of ourselves and what we do.*
3. *Some of us have buddies who have agreed to observe how we work with patients with a stoma.*
4. *Support from the unit/ward leaders and surgeons.*

Challenge:
1. *We need honest, open and constructive feedback about our work with these patients and their spouses, partners and families.*
2. *We need to ask each other questions that make us think about what we just take for granted.*
3. *The patients who join our mini-project team will give us feedback on our actions at each group session.*

Desired outcomes for workplace culture (see person-centred template)

Patient/spouse/partner/family outcomes:

Feel valued as a person and that their beliefs, values and needs as they see them are being considered by the multi-professional team.
Feel more engaged in relationships with multi-professional team members
Feel they are sharing in decision-making about stoma care and adjustment

Multi-professional team outcomes:

Knowing self – more self-aware
More thoughtful/reflective about service they offer
Effective interpersonal skills
Shared decision-making between patients, spouses, partners or family members and the team

Ward/unit outcomes:

Contributing to the creation of a person-centred culture in the ward/unit
More empowered patients/spouses/partners and team
Person-centred ward rounds

Chart: What activities do I/we need to undertake to achieve my/our objective? (Note: one chart for each objective)

Key activity	Timescale for activity (start/end dates)	Lead and key stakeholders, participants	Stakeholders I/we will account to about my/our work
Feedback the plan to the practice development group	5 October	Ann – lead	Practice development group
Put up a poster about the project on the ward noticeboard and in the day room inviting patients, and if they so wish, their spouses, partners, family members to attend a session to explain the project and invite them to participate in it. Similar poster in the surgeons' office inviting them to participate.	15 October – 8 November	Mary – lead Fiona & Margaret	Patients with a stoma, spouses, partners, family members, practice development group, unit/ward leaders, multi-professional team colleagues
Ask for a slot at the buddy training sessions for the following: • introduce the project • talk about how staff behaviours can disempower patients with a stoma and make them feel worthless, disown their stoma and delay or prevent their adjustment to living with a stoma	2 October – 18 December	Jan – Lead John & Colleen	
• discuss what the baseline evidence shows in terms of the multi-professionals' behaviour and relationships with patients with a stoma • get staff commitment to the project			↓
Practise new skills in helping patients look after their own stomas, own their stoma and adjust to living with it. Ask buddy to observe and vice versa and give each other constructive feedback	2 October – 1 February	Ann – Lead All project group members and their buddies	Buddy
Model (show others) new behaviours and person-centred partnerships with patients with a stoma. We also model how to challenge colleagues if they revert to old behaviours and non-person-centred relationships with patients.	1 February – 1 October	Fiona – lead All project group members	Patients with a stoma, spouses, partners, family members, practice development group, unit/ward leaders, multi-professional team colleagues
Repeat the baseline evaluation (patient stories and observations of care) in the middle and at the end of the project (when patients attend 3 and 9 month out-patient follow-up appointments). Write up a short project report and circulate it to all stakeholders including the Executive team of the hospital. Discuss submitting a paper about the project to the International Practice Development Journal (www.fons.org)	1 April & 30 September	John – lead Helen & Martin	↓

- **What evidence will I/we need to have to evaluate the achievement of the objectives? (Refer back to desired outcomes with workplace culture.)**
- **What methods and criteria for success will I/we use to evaluate the achievement of the key activities and objectives?**
- **Who will help to check that the evidence does show that achievement?**

We will need to repeat the patient stories and observations of care to document the presence or absence of person-centred, enabling care of patients with a stoma and their spouses, partners or family members and also ask patients to give us feedback on an ongoing basis if they are willing and able to.

Criteria for success will be:

All patients with a stoma will be offered help by the ward nursing team to look after their own stomas.

The multi-professional team members will create the conditions for patients with stomas to ask questions and raise their concerns during everyday care and on ward rounds.

Who needs to know about the action plan (e.g. stakeholders, managers)?

Practice development group, the multi-professional team, unit and ward leaders, patients, spouses, partner or family members, stoma care community nurses, hospital chaplain.

How will I/we evaluate our learning about practice development and workplace culture?

We will review and evaluate each project group session meeting, ward round and the work we do with our buddies to:

- *examine the ways we are relating to patients, the multi-professional team, project stakeholders and whether there is evidence that we are becoming more person-centred within the project*
- *explore whether what we are learning in terms of person-centred care of patients with a stoma is spilling over into other aspects of our work*
- *identify the practice development processes and methods we are using, how effectively we are using them and whether they are helping us to contribute to the development of a person-centred workplace culture in the ward and unit.*

Date action plan agreed
Insert date: _____

PRACTICE DEVELOPMENT participants' names:
(All names)

_____
_____
_____
_____
_____

Key milestones and target dates
Year 1

Activity/milestone	Lead	Target date	Comments about achievement and progress
Each member of the ward nursing team has worked alongside a colleague who has modelled how to support patients with a stoma	MW	1 Jan	
All patients with a stoma are offered support with managing their own stoma and with owning, and coming to terms with, their stoma by members of the multi-disciplinary team	JS	1 Oct	
We hear staff recognising when they are engaging in non-person-centred behaviours and challenging others (in supportive ways) when we observe or experience others behaving in non-person-centred ways	JS	1 Oct	

What do you do with this next?

If you work in a care setting that hasn't been involved in mini-projects before or with working with key stakeholders to develop practice, you might find it helpful to look back at previous chapters of this resource and refresh your memory on how to work in collaborative, inclusive and participative ways. For example, in chapters 2–5, there are many group activities. Look at them again, this time with an eye to the kinds of things we suggest the facilitator can do. Chapter 8 is likely to be an important resource for you in terms of learning how to be more reflective and evaluative about your own contribution to the project as a leader/participant. It could also be useful in helping you to enable group working that produces the desired outcomes and, at the same time, helps everyone to learn and become more person-centred and effective, not only in the project but also in daily work.

Chapter 8 Learning in the Workplace

Contents

Introduction

Learning in the workplace is a very important feature of developing your workplace culture. Everything we do in practice development to promote person-centred workplace culture will involve learning and evaluation about:

- yourself and the impact you have on others;
- yourself and the level to which you enable others to have an impact on you;
- how to do something new, change practice and workplace cultures;
- whether you have been effective in doing these things and whether they have made a different to those who work and receive care in your care setting and to people who visit in the setting.

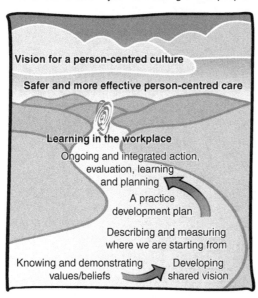

Fig. 8.1 The next step: Learning in the workplace.

Practice Development Workbook for Nursing, Health and Social Care Teams, First Edition. Jan Dewing, Brendan McCormack, and Angie Titchen.
© 2014 John Wiley & Sons, Ltd. Published 2014 by John Wiley & Sons, Ltd.
Companion website: www.wiley.com/go/practicedevelopment/workbook

There is material in this chapter that will be useful to all team members. This material helps people to learn from their work whilst they are actually in the workplace. Much of the material, however, is aimed at those leading, coordinating and facilitating the practice development. There are guides that will help those people to understand how to facilitate the creation of a person-centred learning environment, promote active learning and offer learning supervision. This work is not extra – it can be done through the activities of the practice development itself. This understanding is likely to help them to be able to introduce and point out relevant activities and tools to the rest of the team.

Up until now, this workbook has taken you on the practice development journey towards a better workplace culture and at the same time helping you to learn in the workplace either on your own or with others. In this chapter, we will build on the learning processes we have introduced you to so far. In addition, we show you how having a learning culture at work makes developing practice easier to achieve. There are fundamental differences between a learning environment and a learning culture, which we will explore in this chapter. However, you might like to reflect on what these might be.

In Chapter 4, we said that structured reflection is vital and the team members need to be reflective, evaluating their own feelings, motivations and actions. If this does not happen then it is unlikely that the vision of a person-centred workplace culture will be fully achieved. This also means that person-centred care will not be achieved. Imagine how difficult it would be to progress along the path if stakeholders did not reflect on and learn from the findings of the baseline evaluation? How could a plan be made to address unsatisfactory aspects of care, the service setting or home life unless people reflect on what it is that makes it unsatisfactory? How could mini-projects be set up, for example, to redress the lack of power that many patients/residents and families have in health care or in running of the care setting, or to redress the feeling that their personal identity has been taken away? Unless team members unite and engage around common needs, progress will be slow or impossible.

As a recap, practice development is based on the idea that you/we need to reflect on, and come to understand, ourselves and what is happening before you/we can change anything significantly. And that understanding usually comes through taking things apart and putting them back together in new ways. New understanding will inform our actions to change yourself, our practices and the care setting. Sometimes new understanding emerges through generating new ways of doing things (i.e. innovating) that appear to work but we don't know why. Stopping to reflect at that point increases understanding. This latter option suits people who don't have a great need to take things apart to understand there is a need to change; they just want to get on with the process of doing something.

Look now at the practice development framework (Figure 1.2) that we set out in Chapter 1 of this workbook. Relevant to you for this chapter is 'Learning together'; by changing yourself and your setting, you will help create the person-centred learning culture as seen in the middle of the diagram.

Many people equate learning at work with training; for example, being sent on a course or attending study days or practical updating sessions. If you have done some of the activities in this workbook, you will know by now that learning at work is much more than that. In this chapter, we expand and deepen the ways in which you can learn from your work, with your learning buddy and with others including patients/residents and families by introducing you to the idea of *active learning* (Dewing, 2007, 2008a). We also look at active learning in a more *formal learning relationship* with a *facilitator*, *supervisor* or *critical friend* and point you in the direction of other resources that may be useful to you here. The focus is on active learning supported by the clinical leader or manager and/or others in our care setting who are already in facilitation of learning roles and can also offer informal help in the midst of everyday practice. We also show you some of the ways that you can make a care setting or home a good place to learn in for everyone who works and lives there.

The principles of active learning are:

- dialogue with self through different modes of reflection (e.g. written, drawing, painting, poetic, walks);
- dialogue or structured conversation with others (i.e. more than simply 'chat');
- seeing and doing in the workplace;
- trying out or experimenting with new ways of offering care and working in the team;
- evaluation of achievements in the workplace and of learning.

You might be able to see now that we have been encouraging active learning methods throughout this resource.

Central to creating a person-centred (learning) culture and to practice development work is giving others effective feedback (as you have seen in Chapter 5 when giving feedback from your observations of care and the workplace). Also central is posing effective questions that encourage the other person's learning. Such feedback and questions help people to become more effective as an individual and when working with others. This effectiveness is essential for being person-centred with patients/residents, families and fellow team workers. However, in order to offer or give feedback you must also be prepared to receive it from others.

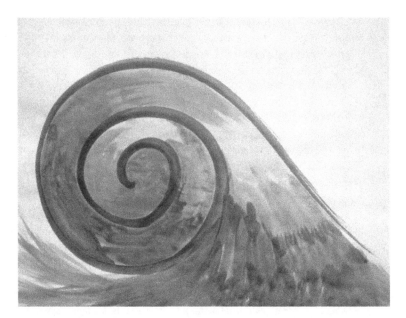

Fig. 8.2 Just as spirals are found all around us in nature, facilitation and learning are often depicted by practice developers as spirals.

Skilled practice developers use multiple methods to enable building up a culture where giving and receiving feedback and asking questions becomes an everyday activity, both formally and informally. Examples of informal feedback dialogues include conversations between team members and patients/residents relating to satisfaction and evaluation of care/service, or team members talking about an aspect of their practice. Examples of more formal giving and receiving of feedback include structured and facilitated encounters in practice development groups, mini-project groups, stakeholder and team sessions and even in meetings.

Resources in this chapter

The resources are set out in three parts: Creating a person-centred learning environment (culture and infrastructure that supports learning), Active learning and Learning supervision. There are Frequently Asked Questions in Chapter 9 *When learning in the workplace gets underway (which should be all the way along the practice development journey!)* that are relevant to this chapter.

Part 1: Creating a person-centred learning environment

- **A learning infrastructure and culture guide and activity** – the guide suggests what you might expect to see in a care setting that is committed to creating a learning *culture* and *infrastructure* for team members, patients/residents and families. The activity helps you to make a comparison with your own care setting/home.
- **A framework for work-based learning** (Manley et al., 2009) (available on companion website) – work-based learning is about learning in and from work through programmes of support offered by a partnership between an education provider, an employee and the employing organisation. This framework is also relevant for learning in and from work where there is no such partnership. The framework points out the things that help learning in the workplace (i.e. a learning culture and supportive care setting infrastructure). It shows the features of a setting/home that would indicate that learning happens and is supported in the workplace (e.g. active learners, learning from and with others, and everyday work as the basis for learning). The framework also highlights the consequences of work-based learning (e.g. individual/team effectiveness and patients/residents benefitting from the team learning). You can see this resource on the publisher's website (**www.wiley.com/go/practicedevelopment/workbook**).

- **Activities and guidance for creating a person-centred, learning environment** – here we offer activities and guidance (using processes that you are probably becoming familiar with or are quite familiar with now) to start getting into place the things that will help effective work-based learning to happen. The central role of the clinical leader/ manager in leading and supporting this work is reflected in the activities. We include a resource on evaluation and process review of sessions to help you learn how to be more effective, not only in planning and contributing to sessions, but also how to use them as a method to enable learning that will help create and sustain a person-centred, learning culture (**www.wiley.com/go/practicedevelopment/workbook**).

- **Giving and receiving feedback effectively** – this is a powerful force for transformation, but if it is ineffective, it can be quite the opposite. Introducing feedback in a culture where feedback is currently experienced as threatening or blaming, needs special attention to be paid to introducing and nurturing it in constructive and safe ways. This group of materials takes the form of handouts or cue sheets and describes some of the central indicators you can use when you put together and offer feedback to others and when you introduce it. The indicators of effective and ineffective feedback can be found on the companion website (**www.wiley.com/go/practicedevelopment/workbook**) and you can use that resource as a cue sheet for yourself to enable you to evaluate the feedback you receive from others to see how well put together it is. You can adapt these indicators to the feedback situation (the context) you are in, the amount of time you have and whether the feedback is planned or unplanned. Used as handouts for others, these materials can promote a discussion about what feedback is and isn't and its purpose in practice development. Groups, for example mini-project groups, can use these handouts to help generate their own ground rules for giving and receiving feedback.

- **Questions to enable increased awareness, reflection and action** – asking effective questions is another core skill for a practice developer to have and to continually nurture. We include two resources here, *Questions that can be used with Giving and receiving feedback* and *Enabling questions*. The questions in the reflection tools in the companion website are also worth revisiting, as they offer numerous effective questions that can be used in a range of practice development scenarios (such as one-to-one dialogues with your buddy, supervisor, group discussions and working with patients/residents and families). It is essential to know what questions to ask and when to ask them. Thus, having a 'bank' of effective questions can be worthwhile investing in.

    Effective questions are those which:
    - help clarify the subject or topic – they are necessary before using reflective questions (clarification questions are ones that aid your understanding of a situation or its context but do not usually require an in-depth answer from another person);
    - help you or another person to expand the way you or they think and feel;
    - enable others to want to engage in solving a puzzle or issue;
    - ultimately enable action in the workplace that will increase effectiveness in person-centred practice.

Part 2: Active learning

- **Activities and guidance for facilitating active learning** – this section offers a guide for asking enabling questions, and a range of activities. The activities include practising the use of enabling questions, reflecting on and evaluating yourself as an active learner and examining the way you reflect. There is an activity to show you how to do a 15 minute reflection in the working day, another to help you to help others reflect by focusing on positive incidents and, finally, an activity using a straightforward tool to solve problems effectively alone and with others.

- **Worksheet for recording learning and action points** – a simple tool to help you record what you have learned from any kind of learning event, for example a reflection, discussion or workshop. You can either photocopy a number of sheets to keep a learning record over time or, once you are familiar with it, you can use the elements of the tool in your learning notebook to save on photocopying. Check first to see whether your organisation has a standard template that you are already asked to use.

- **Resources for learning about active learning processes** – this comprises a series of simple resources that can be used as part of active learning that you do with your buddy (or facilitator, supervisor or critical friend) or they can be used at shift handover, team sessions, practice development groups, mini-project sessions or sessions with stakeholders. In all these contexts they can be used for your own learning as an active learner, to share with others if you are a group leader, facilitator, supervisor or critical friend, or for evaluation, including:
    - process evaluation: listening critically;
    - process evaluation record: listening skills;
    - process evaluation record: what I said.

    Then there is an evaluation tool to evaluate active learning. The tool is intended for use at the end of an active learning session, but that doesn't mean it needs to be used at the end of every session. However, periodic use is good for capturing evidence over time.

Part 3: Learning supervision

- **Induction programmes, preceptorship, mentorship, coaching and work-based learning facilitation** – these types of learning supervision are briefly described so that the differences and overlaps between them are clear.

- **Guide for work-based facilitators: foundation degrees** – this is an excerpt from Canterbury Christ Church University materials that explains what work-based learning is when there is a partnership between an education provider (in this case, the university) and employers and employees.
- **Clinical supervision for the future** – for team and clinical leaders interested in developing clinical supervision for team members, we present a link to a resource that could help get things started.
- **Summary of learning in the workplace** – a concluding summary is offered.

PART 1: Creating a person-centred learning environment (culture and infrastructure that supports learning)

We suggest that in Part 1, all care team members will find the learning culture guide helpful. Also, the handout on giving and receiving feedback is likely to be useful, either all of it or at least the activity at the beginning of the handout. The rest of Part 1 will help those leading, coordinating and facilitating the practice development to create a culture and infrastructure in the care setting or home that will support learning in the workplace. The material will help them to explain to the team members what a person-centred learning environment is.

Sheet 8.1: A learning culture guide

This guide is for all the team members. It sets out the kinds of things you would expect to see, hear and feel as you walk about a care setting that is committed to developing a learning culture for team members and for the people who receive care or live there as well as families.

You might like to watch one or more of these videos first:

Art for their sake In 1978, George Nicholas (an artist and cartoonist from Liverpool) and a community arts team 'Art For Their Sake' offered their services as muralists free of charge to Alder Hey Children's Hospital in Merseyside. Imagine how their creation might contribute towards a learning environment in a hospital. (www.youtube.com/watch?v=Ph4iMdMIfVY&feature=related)

She without arm, he without leg Imagine what it took for the two dancers to learn a new way of dancing. Are there any insights for you as a person in the process of becoming facilitator of workplace learning? (www.youtube.com/watch?v=UTrb6i7gJAk&hd=1)

Where the hell is Matt? What does this say about the qualities of being a facilitator of work-based learning? What are the processes going on? (www.youtube.com/watch?v=zlfKdbWwruY)

Personalisation for older people: Residential care This video is an example of a care home that has a well-developed learning culture for residents (as well as team members). You may like to make notes on what you think indicates a person-centred, learning environment. (www.scie.org.uk/socialcaretv/video-player.asp?guid=6848a684-1ef3-4e7c-9c32-a3f029717d93)

Commentary

The key indication of a person-centred learning culture in this video is the importance the care setting places on getting to know the resident as a person with a history, background and particular things they like to do, as the starting point for treating each resident as an individual. There is a focus in their work with people with dementia to help them relearn who they are. For instance, knowing that Marjorie used to play the organ in her local church and that music was (and still is) an important part of her life, they sit with her at the keyboard for a very short period each day to help her relearn her favourite hymns. Achievement is rewarded, 'Encore!'.

And feedback on the effectiveness is sought. 'If you say something that resonates with the person, you will get a recognition, feedback, a smile'. Did you see that feedback when 'The Mallard' train was placed in Roger's hands?

In this home, relatives are also helped to learn, for example, to live with difficult, painful feelings like the 'giving up' up on their family member when they are admitted or getting through their first Christmas after the death of their loved one. Did you notice the care workers 'being with' people, like sitting at the table with them (when it was not a mealtime). Such opportunities open the way for learning about the person and how to strive for their well-being through a person-centred relationship.

Information-giving

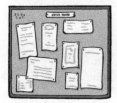

Here are some other things you might see or hear in a care setting with a person-centred learning culture.

- *General noticeboards and leaflets* for all team members, patients/residents and families, which could include:
  - the ward/unit/clinic/care home vision statements;
  - general information about the ward or department and who works there
    - name of nurse/midwife or therapist in charge;
    - an explanation of what different uniforms and colours mean;
  - quality reports with metrics and other quality data;
  - practice development posters, evaluation and progress updates on mini-projects;
  - notification of stakeholder meetings;
  - notification of open educational events being held in the care setting, for example about person-centred practice or using information technology (IT);
  - personal development events and opportunities beyond the workplace, for example learning a second language, keep fit classes, chair exercise group, open access courses on the Internet, learning how to communicate anywhere in the world for free on the Internet;
  - news items about, and photos of, people living there;
  - leaflets about person-centred care and issues relevant to team members and people living there;
  - useful website details and resources;
  - agendas and notes of meetings of the Practice Development Coordinating group;
  - public library access and hospital/care home 'library' services;
  - links to local specialists and community education;
  - contact names, for example IT support, booking spaces/rooms for groups and meetings, learning champion, hospital/care home 'library', activities coordinator.

  Noticeboards and leaflets for patients and families could include:
  - information on how to make a compliment/accolade or a complaint;
  - social and community notices;
  - training, learning and development information aimed at patients and families;
  - a vision statement about the learning environment.
- Learning and social opportunities/activities for older people and families offered in the care home or local community by volunteers, community groups or the University of the Third Age (www.u3a.org.uk/), for example participative, interactive drama groups, book club, cookery, gardening, artwork, collage-making, quilting, chess, local history, current affairs:
  - information about invited speakers and talks;
  - leaflets on local social services, self-help groups, community groups (actual and virtual (i.e. on the Internet));
  - social activities, e.g. films, quizzes, dances;
  - social citizen group activities for local, national and international campaigns relating to issues important to older people and their families, e.g. protecting wildlife, climate change, older people's rights, raising funds.
- *Noticeboards and leaflets for team members* could include:
  - a vision statement about the learning environment for team members;
  - information about what support for learning the care setting/home offers team members, e.g. clinical supervision, mentorship, critical friends, individual learning and development plans, a buddy system and training, 15 minute reflection spaces, positive incident accounts and development planning;
  - timetable for agreeing individual learning and development plans and meetings with buddy/supervisor;
  - invitations from members of the team to share their learning and new skills with fellow workers;
  - an invitation for nominations for learning champions (members who spread the word about the benefits of learning and development and run 'drop in' sessions);
  - information about educational frameworks and opportunites, e.g. National Vocational Qualifications, foundation degrees;
  - short accounts of successes and achievements of team members who are putting their learning into practice and how they are making a difference.

Thanks for this invitation to comment on the idea of setting up a Practice Development Coordination Group. I think it is an excellent idea as it will make the development work more efficient.

As someone who is frequently re-admitted to the ward, I would like to offer my services as a group member.

Amelia

Collaboration, Inclusion and Participation (CIP)

- Interactive boards (these might be a section on any of the above noticeboards) inviting responses to any current issue in the care setting/home (pads of sticky notes could be attached to the boards).

Other things you might see and hear (depending on the type of care setting) might be:

- newspapers and magazines;
- bookshelves with large print books and audio books;
- computers with easy access;
- service/home manager:
    - inquiring about team members' learning;
    - acknowledging and celebrating team members' achievements;
    - sharing staff achievements with others;
    - holding coffee mornings for questions and answers about the practice development;
    - patient/resident groups or committees;
    - family groups or committees.

Team members (including service/home care managers), patients/residents and families:

- evaluating the care/service just given/event experienced, sharing what they have learned from the care/service given and agreeing action point plans based on that learning (e.g. productive series information);
- giving each other helpful feedback during the course of daily work;
- rehearsing a dance or inter-generational drama performance with local school children;
- sharing new ideas with each other;
- asking each other questions to help the other person to reflect more deeply;
- offering high challenge and high support to each other;
- staff accompanying a resident on an outing;
- celebrating success and rewarding people for trying.

Team members:

- sitting and learning together in short reflective spaces in the working day;
- using a variety of processes at the end of handover and meetings to evaluate effectiveness;
- sitting with a patient/resident asking about their views or experience on a specific topic.

Sheet 8.2: Activity and guidance for managers for creating a person-centred learning environment

The central role of the care setting manager in leading and supporting development work is reflected in this activity. Whilst the activity and guide are intended for the manager (or a person in a similar role), other team members who are leading, coordinating or facilitating change may also find it useful.

This activity uses the framework for work-based learning (available on the companion website). Using processes that you are probably quite familiar with now, the activity will help you start thinking about how you could get the enabling factors and attributes of work-based learning into place.

As the manager, you know that you are responsible for setting and leading the strategic direction and that this should include learning. It is commonly accepted that the leader or manager leads on creating a learning culture and setting up a supportive infrastructure for learning in the workplace. This is not to say that you, as manager, have to do all the work of creating a person-centred learning environment. As with all the practice development work, it is likely that you will be taking a lead role on enabling stakeholders to contribute to the work. In addition, you are in an ideal position to model being a practitioner in such an environment and learning from your own work.

We invite you to ask yourself, and then reflect on, the following questions:

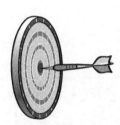

- Are the enabling factors of a context-wide learning culture and supportive infrastructure in place?
- If yes,
  - Referring to what I have learned about creating person-centred, learning cultures and supportive infrastructures through using this resource, are the enabling factors fully in place to support the attributes of work-based learning?
  - Are the attributes of learning in the workplace relevant to the care setting/home and if so, are they clearly visible?
    - What is an active learner?
    - Is everyday work the focus for learning in the home?
    - Are sufficient resources available?
    - Are the systems in place and working well?
  - Do any of the attributes fall short and need my attention?
- If no,
  - How can I use what I have learned from this resource to work towards getting these enabling factors and attributes in place?
  - How can I involve stakeholders in getting them into place?
  - Are there any other resources that I could tap into for inspiration for this work?

Guidance

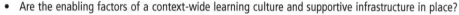

1. Thinking back to any of the activities in Chapters 2 and 3 of this workbook, that you, team members, patients/residents and families undertook, you will remember that it is our values and beliefs that shape the workplace cultures we create, so:
   - were any values and beliefs brought to the surface around how to achieve person-centred practice that you could build on?
   - were any of these values and beliefs relevant to learning in the workplace?
     - if so, could you use the team's *values clarification* work to remind them that learning at work is vital to the success of the person-centred workplace culture?
     - if not, is another values clarification activity around learning in the workplace necessary? Or a *Claims, Concerns and Issues* about learning opportunities in the working day?

2. Now recall any *activities* you have undertaken in this resource or sessions you have called or attended in relation to the practice development:
   - were there any opportunities for you to:
     - encourage team/patient/resident/family member learning or reflection;
     - ask them about their learning;
     - offer high challenge with high support;
     - acknowledge their learning and the impact it has had;
     - give them feedback about their work;
     - celebrate their learning and share it with others;
     - model your own learning at work, acknowledge when you could have done things better, show them how you reflect on and evaluate your own daily work, then develop learning and action points from your reflection and evaluation?
3. Think about your daily work:
   - do you intentionally model person-centred care for team members?
   - do you actively seek the above opportunities to promote reflection and learning and maximise talent within your everyday activities by:
     - negotiating with team members who want to learn from their daily work that you will help them by seizing the moment in whatever is happening at the time;
     - observing, listening, smelling, feeling what is going on and then finding a non-threatening private, informal opportunity to give feedback or high challenge/high support (see handout on Giving and receiving feedback in this chapter);
     - using public corridor conversations and coffee/tea breaks to praise team members/patients/residents and family members for achievements and learning, give general team feedback;
     - building the above opportunities into formalised individual learning and development plans with team members
       - do you help them to identify their potential and learning needs?
   - do you offer people personal learning opportunities to achieve their potential?

Example 1

You are working at the computer in the ward nursing station and you see a nurse and a physiotherapist come into the station. They are talking about 'a problematic neck breather'.

Imagine the conversation then goes something like this:

You look up and say 'Hello, Denise and Sally, how are you doing, both of you?' They both smile and acknowledge you.

You go on to to say 'Are you talking about Linda McGrath when you say, "problematic neck breather"?' They nod, 'Yes'.

You go on, 'I was asking because, as you know, we are trying to create a person-centred culture on the ward. We have all signed up to not labelling patients. I know that it is difficult to change long-standing, non-person-centred language, so I'd really like your help here . . . what do you think is the effect of labelling Linda in this way? What does it say about our ward culture? I know you are busy now, but would it be worth reflecting on this, and perhaps we could have a brief conversation about it over coffee tomorrow with whoever else is around?'

Thus, you have modelled person-centred behaviour in your interaction with Denise and Sally. You have empathised and not attached any blame as you offered them the feedback. You have also suggested that they and other team members consider whether they would like to explore this any further.

Example 2

You might be walking through the home to see an older person and you overhear two members of the team referring to the person as 'a troublemaker'. Later that day, in a private moment, you feed back to the two team members what you heard. You begin by saying 'I heard you refer to Mr D as . . . I would like to ask you whether you were aware that you were referring to Mr D in this way?'

After the responses you say 'I want to invite you both to reflect on this and what it says about your values. I will come back and we can discuss this later today.'

(Note: leaving some space and time for reflection is vital – this encourages team members to work things out for themselves and avoids them being told the answer or what to do.)

Then when you return, you ask the team members how they might feel if someone used such language about them.

You ask the team members how this terminology sits with the shared values and vision the team have signed up to and remind them, in a supportive way, that it has been agreed by everyone in the home that disrespectful language should not be used.

You empathise and do not attach any blame as you give the feedback.

You may want to suggest that the team members consider whether they need help and support to better understand this person's needs.

Before embarking on the practice development journey, you and key stakeholders may have concluded that the strategic direction and strategic plans for the home were sufficient for achieving a person-centred culture. If you have reflected on the questions and guidance above, you and the key stakeholders might decide now to revisit the strategic plans to ensure that there is explicit provision for the enabling factors for promoting work-based learning.

4. Do you have any learning needs around leading on learning? If you do, you may find the *Leading on Learning: A hands-on guide for line managers* publication helpful. This is a great little booklet for leaders, with lots of good ideas for helping managers to promote a learning culture in the workplace. You can download it for free. (www.campaign-for-learning.org.uk/cfl/assets/documents/Informationandfacts/Line%20Managers%20booklet.pdf)

   There are other resources on the Campaign for Learning website such as networking, projects and research that you might find useful too.

5. Do you have any learning needs around facilitating learning in your workplace? If yes, then the rest of this chapter is for you.

Sheet 8.3: Evaluation and process review of group work and sessions

This resource is suitable for team members and those who lead or are members of work groups, such as mini-project teams, coordinating groups, learning groups or the overall practice development coordination group. It is also suitable for learning buddies.

We have already pointed out the idea of summarising key learning and action points that come out of a session or discussion of any kind. In this resource, we show how you can make your sessions more effective by doing a quick evaluation of how they went. From time to time, you may also choose to conduct this activity as a 'process review' as well to learn in more detail what works and what doesn't work in terms of making the discussion effective and a learning opportunity. Thus, these activities support person-centred infrastructures and learning cultures.

Quick evaluation

At the end of each group session, simply asking people how things went is a form of evaluation. There a number of simple and fast ways you can choose and vary to establish how effective your working together was. For example:

1. Ask each person to say briefly what:
   • they liked most;
   • they liked least;
   • they learned.
2. On a sticky note:
   score from 1–10 high challenge:
   a. received by you from others;
   b. given to others by you.
   Score from 1–10 on high support:
   c. received by you from others;
   d. given to others by you.
3. Ask 'What is better about the session?' This can produce positive evaluations.
4. Do a Claims, Concerns and Issues activity about the session.
5. Ask each person to capture the essence of their experience or what they have learned in one to three words. . . . For example, *'motivating'*, *'hopeful'*, *'unsure at this point'*.
6. Invite people to pick a picture card or postcard that best symbolises what they have learned about themselves and the way the group is working.
7. If you want to get really creative, ask them, e.g. what colour the learning was or whether the meeting was a song/ TV show/garden, what would it be?

Remember to keep the comments focused and record the evaluations, so you can learn from them and mark your progress over time towards being person-centred and effective. You do not do all of these – just choose which one works for your purposes.

It is important to remember that the evaluation is not an opportunity to open up a discussion – unless time has been set aside for this to happen. Neither should people go back into items already discussed or try to bring up something new to discuss.

Process review

A process review gives you more detailed information and helps you to learn about how effective your skills are as a buddy, group/team lead or member. Doing a process review is where the observation and listening skills you may have gained in gathering evidence for the development of the practice development plan comes in handy!

Before you begin, everyone in the group or you and your buddy need to agree to doing a process review and what the focus should be. It is a good idea to agree a focus, for example respectfulness, facilitation/reflection skills, the kinds of questions that people ask, whether action plans are revisited and worked on or whether people are listening to or actively engaged with each other. You may agree also to make some very brief notes or scribble down key words about what happens in relation to the focus during the meeting.

Remember, you are still taking part in the session or group, so this is a step up from being a 'fly on the wall' type of observer as it is more difficult to do two things at once. If you are working in a larger group and have decided to have more than one focus, then you might split the things up, so, for example, one person is observing and listening to the person who is facilitating the group, someone else is listening to the questions that anyone asks and how they are asked and someone else is observing and listening to the interactions that happen in the meeting. You may find it helpful to make yourself an observation 'template' for taking a few notes and capturing any insights that you have.

At the end, the person leading the group invites feedback about what has been observed or heard. If you did observations of care/the workplace for the baseline evaluation, you will remember, in Chapter 5, that we stressed the importance of giving others feedback in a challenging but supportive way. We build on the materials offered there about feedback just below.

After the feedback, the group lead/facilitator helps everyone to identify:

- what they have learned from the feedback;
- what they did well and why;
- how they could build on that;
- what they could do better and why;
- how they could do it better.

Group learning points and action points are agreed and recorded for review in a specified time period.

This next resource is a handout that you can use with the team to discuss and prepare for building up the giving and receiving of feedback in your team and workplace.

Sheet 8.4: Giving and receiving feedback handout

Giving and receiving feedback is essential to creating a person-centred learning culture. So the information in this handout is for all team members. It is important to get this message about feedback across in the right way for people, so if you are a leader, coordinator or facilitator in developing practice you might think it best to modify the handout. For example, you might only use parts of it to make it simpler or change the words to language that is right for the team members. On the other hand, you may feel it best to talk team members through the information here, again in language they are familiar with.

This handout and the cue sheets about indicators of effective and ineffective feedback (see companion website) can promote a discussion about what feedback is and isn't and its purpose in practice development. Groups, for example mini-project groups, can use these materials to help to generate their own ground-rules for giving and receiving feedback.

If we are going to develop person-centred infrastructures and learning cultures, we need to be open to receiving feedback from fellow workers about how they see and experience our work. We also need to take the risk of giving fellow workers feedback about what we have observed. Communication of feedback needs to be based on mutual trust, openness and honesty. In turn, this means that we have to be able to offer clear and useful feedback to the people we work with and also ensure that they can offer it to us.

Example

You are working with a colleague and you notice that they did not involve Alex, a young man with a learning difficulty in the decisions about his day. Later, in a private, quiet moment, you ask, in a supportive way whether you can offer some feedback. You stress that your feedback is given as an opportunity for learning and not for blame or criticism. You say that you saw they cut short Alex's attempt to say what he wanted to do that day. You ask them whether they were aware of doing that and what was going on for them at that time. This gives a 'face-saving' opportunity, that is, the chance to say that they know they didn't get it right and probably to offer a reason why.

If it isn't mentioned, you make a link to the behaviour you saw and the values that have been agreed by all of you that the young people in the house should be helped to have a share in decisions about their day. You empathise with how difficult it is to do this in the moment and when it's busy, and you stress that it does make a difference to do it. You do not attach any blame as you give the feedback. You offer space for a response. You do not tell them what to do or how to do it.

Giving and receiving feedback

Effective facilitation relies on communication with groups and with individuals. Communication in facilitation needs to be based on openness and honesty. In turn, this means that effective facilitation requires us to be able to offer clear and useful feedback to the people we work with and also to ensure that they can offer it to us. This can take place in formal situations – supervision for example – or informal settings – for example, as a consequence of a particular incident.

Activity Think of times when you have been given feedback. What, in your experience, makes feedback useful? And, what kind of feedback is unhelpful? What could the other person have done differently? How could you have behaved differently? Make some brief notes as you could use your reflections to help you and others develop your own principles for giving and receiving feedback.

The purpose of feedback

In facilitation we emphasise the importance of facilitation as a means of helping people to learn. An important factor in motivating people is ensuring that they receive feedback that both challenges and supports them, that is, that helps people to see what they are doing well and the effects it has, as well as understanding how they could develop their skills and knowledge further.

Giving feedback: What works

No matter how far you have developed your skills, offering and receiving feedback may cause some discomfort for one or both parties. It is not always possible to prepare to offer or receive feedback, but if you can prepare, it is a valuable way to provide an opportunity to stand back from a situation. The person providing feedback has the opportunity to structure what they want to say, while the person receiving it has a chance to carry out a self-assessment (whether using a framework, or thinking about a particular situation).

The intention of feedback is always to help another person be more effective in their work with patients/residents, families, visitors and co-workers. To this end, thought needs to be given to choosing the right place (thinking about privacy and calmness, for example) and time (in the event of debriefing an incident this should be as soon as possible after the event – and try to be able to give the time required rather than rushing off). The content of feedback is important:

- balance – offer positive as well as critical feedback;
- own the feedback – use 'I' statements;
- describe what you have observed rather than judge (i.e. 'I saw . . .', 'I heard . . .');
- be specific rather than making general statements;
- avoid telling the person what to do or what you would do in their position;
- generate and agree ways of addressing the issues raised, although this might need to wait for a follow up discussion as often people need time to absorb what's been said to them.

Giving feedback: What doesn't work

By contrast, feedback that is entirely negative, one-sided, hostile, personal and unexpected is unlikely to have a positive outcome for anyone.

Receiving feedback: What works

Understanding how to receive feedback is important too, both as a means of working effectively yourself and helping colleagues. Some principles to bear in mind include:

- listen – it's too easy to make judgements about what is being said if you have a closed mind;
- avoid arguing, denying, giving extensive explanations, etc.;
- check out anything that you do not understand and ask for specific examples;
- take time with your response rather than reacting straight away, and suggest you meet again;
- where appropriate, consider seeing whether other people would give you similar feedback.

Structured feedback

Models used in practice development can be seen as ways of engaging with structured feedback, for example clinical supervision or reflection on practice. In addition, frameworks such as 360-degree feedback can be used.

Acknowledgement: This handout is adapted from material prepared for the Facilitation in Practice module, Royal Hospitals Trust/University of Ulster, available on the companion website. Please do not modify or reproduce without attributing authorship.

PART 2: Active learning

Part 2 offers you:

- activities and guidance for facilitating active learning;
- a worksheet for recording learning and action points;
- resources for learning about active learning processes.

The materials are useful for all team members to help you become more active learners and/or to facilitate active learning in your teams, work groups and with buddies.

Enabling questions

This guide explains what enabling questions are and what they are not and why and when they are used. It gives some examples of enabling questions to get you started. It is suitable for all care setting team members. It can also be used by leaders, coordinators or facilitators of the practice development to explain what such questions are and to get a discussion going.

Enabling questions are questions that will help you to become more independent and effective learners in your workplace. This is because they help you to go further in the way you think or feel. Then you can use new understandings to develop your workplace or your work more effectively. Enabling questions will help you to learn things for yourself rather than remaining dependent on others to tell you what to do or for advice. Using enabling questions in our daily interactions with team members and older people as well as in active learning sessions (see activity below) will help contribute to creating a person-centred learning environment in the care setting.

Enabling questions encourage reflection and can lead to action. They are open questions in that they do not make any assumptions. Compare, for example, the open, enabling question:

'How do you feel about what happened?'

with the closed question:

'Did that make you feel angry?'

The latter closed question makes the assumption that you felt angry and that you were made to feel in a certain way – as if you had no choices or control. A closed question invites a Yes or No answer and so may not help the person to become reflective. A leading question also tends to invite a Yes or No answer, but it goes further in closing off opportunities for reflection. For example:

'What you did in that situation was inappropriate, wasn't it?'

or

'You should have given that person feedback about their behaviour, shouldn't you?'

Such judgemental and leading questions run the risk of defensive responses. They may also prevent the person exploring the situation, reflecting upon and evaluating their own behaviour and developing action points about how they could behave more effectively in similar situations in the future.

However, when a person has explored, reflected and evaluated for themselves and is still stuck, leading questions can then be used positively as an alternative to merely giving advice. Giving advice is our favourite past-time (and whilst we may be grateful at the time, how often do we take it ourselves?). Examples of advice are

'What you must do first is give that person feedback about their behaviour before going to tell someone else.'

or

'What I have found is that you need to ask patients/residents what they think.'

In coming up with helpful leading questions, you still use your experience to think up the questions, but you are opening up the opportunity for the person to think for themselves and draw their own conclusions. So, you might ask

'In these circumstances, would it be helpful to give that person feedback about their behaviour?'

or

'Have you thought about asking patients/residents what they think?'
'Is . . . a possibility?'

When people begin to be more aware about creating a learning culture and the importance of asking enabling questions, people tend to ask leading questions as they first attempt to help others to learn. These leading questions point others in a direction the questioner believes is the best one. The trick is to try and avoid them (and closed questions and direct advice giving) and build up a bank of enabling questions. It is likely that you will need help to do that and we suggest some ways you can learn with your colleagues in the active learning activities below.

Here are some enabling questions to get you going.

- What could you do . . .?
- It sounds as though you are feeling . . .? Tell me more about it.
- How do you feel . . .?
- What do you think is really going on here?
- What sense are you making of . . .?
- What does . . . mean for you?
- What do you think would happen if . . .?
- Do you think that . . .?
- How would you know if . . .?
- How can you . . .?
- Can we stop for a moment and check on how we are doing?
- How helpful was that comment?
- Perhaps it would be more helpful to turn that comment into a question?
- What question does that raise for you?
- What question was the most helpful?
- Energy levels seem low – shall we take a break?
- Perhaps we should check our agreed ground rules?
- What are we trying to do here?
- How can we help you (or someone else) move forward on this issue?
- How can we make this relationship more effective?
- What does that really mean?
- Are you saying 'they' when you mean 'you'?
- How can I help you?

Don't forget the enabling questions in the reflective tools in Chapter 4 on the companion website.

Activity 8.1: The 15 minute reflection space

> This activity shows how you can use those few precious moments when patients/residents do not need you to better reflect either on your own or with your buddy on something that is happening to you right now and what you can learn from it. This is an activity that every team member can do.

We know that working in health and social care is demanding and that time for reflection is limited. This is why practice developers have developed ways of doing reflection that can be squeezed into most working days. We have suggested, for example, using the shift handover time and corridor conversations for moments of reflection and sharing learning. The 15 minute reflection space is a more formal method that enables a reflective conversation to be carried out with both the person telling their experience and the listener/enabler knowing that they are working to a 15 minute time frame. The method usually follows this process:

> Don't forget to agree ground rules before you begin!

Teller	Gives a quick one liner headline that describes their experience or event (think about this in the form of a newspaper headline)
Helper	Asks for the key points about the headline
Teller	Provides detail in a clear concise way (no more than 3 minutes)
Helper	Asks teller key enabling questions that usually cover some or all of these:
	How did your feelings or other people's, at the time, influence what you did or didn't do?
	How clear were you about the options you had?
	What were the consequences of what you did or didn't do?
	What have you learned from this?
	What will you do differently in the future?
Teller	Responds to each of the enabling questions as they arise
Helper	Brings reflection to a close

An alternative question framework (Fowler et al., 2007) could be:

- So what did it take to do that?
- What helped you to achieve that?
- How did you do that?
- How did you get through that time/experience/deal with that?
- What did you learn about yourself managing to do that?
- What might this have shown others about you?

Activity 8.2: Practising the use of open enabling questions in active learning

This activity is suitable for all team members. Buddies might invite another colleague to join them for the activity, and the facilitator of an active learning group would explain the activity to the group. An active learning group is a small, informal or formal group where one of the group adopts the role of facilitator.

This activity is probably the most important learning activity in Part 2 and it is well worth the time investment.

The purpose of this activity is two-fold: first to help you to practise your enabling questions and second, with others, to do and facilitate active learning more intentionally.

For some years now, we have done this activity (devised originally by McGill and Beaty (2001)) with hundreds of people learning to engage in active learning. What you learn here you can take into shorter time slots of reflection with others in your working day (like the 15 minute reflective space above).

This activity will take 50 minutes with your buddy or 75 minutes in an active learning group. If you are working with your buddy, you might decide to invite a colleague to come and work with you for this activity (in which case it will take 75 minutes so they have a turn too), but you can do it just in your pairs in the 50 minutes.

Key activities

Don't forget to agree ground rules before you begin!

In an active learning group, ask people to organise into sets of threes in the following roles. If you have an even number in the group, the extra person can join a three. With four people there are always two observers. The timing for each presentation is 10 minutes, with 8 minutes for feedback from the observers. If you are doing this with your buddy, the roles are the same but you may or may not have an observer (third person). If you don't, then you will both have to observe yourself and each other as you do the following. Because this is difficult to do, it is best to try to find a third person.

Presenter

You are to think of a task/puzzle/problem/issue about your work or part of the practice development journey and discuss it with one of the group (the enabler). Try to be brief and specific. The 'task', 'puzzle', 'problem' or 'issue' should be of *real* concern to you and not something that you have already developed an answer or response to. It can be anything that matters to you.

Enabler

You are to help the presenter with his or her 'task/puzzle/problem/issue' by trying to get the presenter to think through this in a reflective way. Ask open questions (e.g. How do you know this? What does this mean?). The objective is to enable the presenter to define or redefine their experience and their relationship to it in specific terms so that the *presenter* may be more able to take some steps towards solving it. Try to focus on what can be done *by* the presenter – not what others ought to do and not what you feel would be the right thing to do if it were you or has been you in a similar situation. Some helpful enabling questions* may include:

- What could you do . . .?
- It sounds as though you are feeling . . .? Tell me more about it.
- How do you feel . . .?
- What do you think is really going on . . .?
- What do you think would happen if . . .?
- What is stopping you from . . .?
- How would you know if . . .?
- How can/will you . . .?

Observer

The observer listens to what is being *said or not said*. You observe the verbal interaction and consider what questions/responses were more/less helpful in enabling the presenter to move forward his or her issue. The observer also listens to/senses what the *feelings* of the presenter are in relation to their issue.

Finally, the observer also listens to / senses what the presenter has *invested* (or not) in the issue. What is the presenter's *will, commitment* or *motivation* toward the issue and its possible resolution?

Further points the observer may wish to consider include:

- Is the enabler providing their solutions for the presenter rather than supporting them to work it out for themselves?
- Is the presenter focusing on what they can do rather than what they can't do?
- Is the presenter avoiding resolving the problem?
- Is the presenter's proposed action specific enough?

Take 10 minutes between presenter and enabler (5 minutes each). After the session and a pause, the presenter and enabler (in that order) convey how the experience was for them. The observer then gives feedback for 5 minutes to the 'enabler' on how their facilitation aided the presenter, and to the presenter, and then the presenter and 'enabler' may wish to add their comments.

Change roles, in order that each person can take the role of enabler and presenter.

* Sometimes, the enabler needs to ask some clarifying questions to help the presenter understand the situation, such as 'Who are the key stakeholders involved here?' or 'Had this person already been invited to join the Residents Forum?' Such questions only need short answers. Ask them sparingly because clarifying questions are for you (so you can then ask more effective enabling questions). Be careful that you are not just asking them because you are curious, because they are unlikely to take the other person's understanding further. Don't forget to avoid closed and leading questions because they don't encourage the person to think for themselves. They can really be just another way of telling someone what they could or should do!

Examples of other enabling questions include:

- How do your feelings influence the way you want to act here?
- How can you explore falls with the older person?
- What is stopping you from doing . . .?
- How prepared do you feel?
- How have you secured support for your ideas/plan?

Examples of closed questions include:

- Do you think your negative feelings about the other person are a block? (This is a closed question with an assumed cause included.)
- Can you explore falls in this patient/resident to prevent them from happening? (This is a closed question with an assumed solution included and implies something that will be done to the resident rather than with them.)
- Why don't you tell this person you are going to do . . .? (This is a closed question with a direction or action included.)
- Have you prepared yourself by doing a Claims, Concerns and Issues? (This is a closed question with direction included.)
- Have you asked X to support you with this? (This is a closed question with direction included.)

Sheet 8.5: Preparation for activities 3–6

- Activity 8.3: Reflection on 'self as active learner' (below)
- Activity 8.4: Types/modes of reflection: The way you tend to reflect (available on companion website)
- Activity 8.5: Positive incident accounts (below)
- Activity 8.6: Problem-solving tool (available on companion website)

You can do these activities on your own, with your buddy or in an active learning group.

You will need:

- a reasonably quiet space to reflect in where you will not be interrupted (and that is big enough for the group if that is the way you are working);
- your learning notebook;
- simple creative materials, e.g. cards, coloured pens or pencils.

If you are working with your buddy or a small group, you will also need:

- one of you to facilitate the structure, e.g. ensure that there is a beginning, middle and end to the group work and that everyone has a chance to contribute (see handout on leading a group in Chapter 7;
- everyone in the group to be asking enabling questions (see above) and helping each other to learn.

Key activities

At the beginning of the first activity you do, you need to review any ground rules that you may have developed with your buddy or with the active learning group. You need to ensure that they are sufficient for learning together about learning. Ground rules about giving and receiving feedback are extremely important here. You may already have developed some a while back if you did the activity in Chapter 3 called 'Visioning the practice development processes & developing ground rules'. If you did, check that you included giving and receiving feedback. If you are working now with people who were not involved in the development of those ground rules, then you will need to develop new ones together so that everyone owns them. Everyone might accept the original ground rules, or together you can build on them, changing some bits. Alternatively, you all decide you need new ones. For help with developing them, if necessary, see Part 1 of this chapter, and Chapter 5 in the materials called 'Giving and receiving feedback after evidence gathered'.

At the start of Activities 8.1–8.6, start with an individual reflection. If you are with your buddy or active learning group, take turns to share what you have thought about.

Help each other to go further in your thinking by asking enabling questions (see earlier in this chapter).

Give each other feedback about your learning and celebrate progress.

If you are working in an active learning group, the facilitator leads the turn-taking, asking each other enabling questions, giving feedback and celebrating progress.

Again, don't forget the ground rules!

Activity 8.3: Reflection on 'self as active learner'

This individual activity is one everyone in the team can do. It will help you begin to think about how you are now and your potential as an active learner. It will link back to the reflection tools (available on the companion website) you might have used in Chapter 4.

Ask yourself what you are aware of in relation to:

- your feelings about being an active learner and engaging with the activities in this resource?
- what it means to you to be an active learner?
- the things you take for granted about being an active learner?
- any ideas behind being an active learner?
- the links between the ideas and the values you hold?
- what do I need to do to become a more effective active learner?

If you prefer, you could use one of the reflective tools to think about being an active learner. Check out the companion website (**www.wiley.com/go/practicedevelopment/workbook**).

Now if you are with your buddy or active learning group, follow the key activities set out in the Preparation for Activities 8.3–8.6.

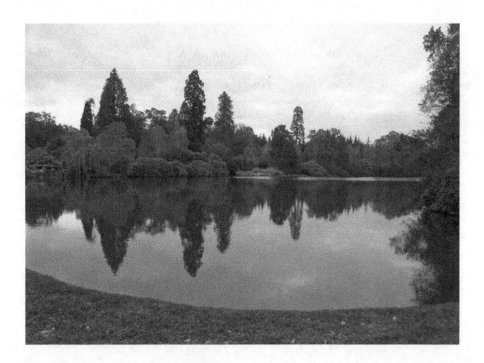

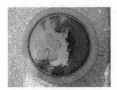

How do you feel when you view this picture? Why do you think we have put it here?

Reflection can take place in multiple ways.

Often, looking at an inspiring photo or painting or other piece of art can either relax the head or stimulate it to reflect. Have you got any photos or paintings you could use in this way? Music can also achieve a similar effect.

Activity 8.5: Positive incident accounts

Positive incident accounts, developed by Jan Dewing, from a project at The Mater Misericordiae University Hospital in Dublin, are essentially about capturing learning from positive events and identifying what you can do with your learning in future similar events or situations. It is aimed at helping you appreciate what is working well and why. It is suitable for all team members.

This activity can be done in 15 minutes on your own, with your buddy or in 30 minutes with an active learning group.

Reflect alone or individually with your buddy or active learning group on something that is going or went really well in the care setting by asking yourself (or your buddy or fellow group member) the following questions (based on Rolfe et al., 2001).

- What is/was it that made this incident so positive?
- What is/was making it possible?
- What are my thoughts, feelings, judgements about the incident / what is/was at the heart of it / what are/were the consequences?
- What ideas do I have about the incident?
- What have I learned from it and how can I use this learning in future in similar situations?
- How can I share this positive account with others?
- How can we celebrate our positive accounts with others?
- How could we build this activity into our daily work?

Now if you are with your buddy or active learning group, follow the key activities as shown earlier in this resource.

Activity 8.6 offers a problem-solving tool that you and your buddy or active learning group may find useful when you are working with something difficult or problematic in a particular situation. It can be found on the companion website at **www.wiley.com/go/practicedevelopment/workbook**.

Sheet 8.6: Worksheet for recording learning and action points

This worksheet is for all team members to use

My learning points

My action points (What specifically will you do?)	Agreed completion date	New skills/knowledge needed? (Detail how these will be acquired)

Sheet 8.7: Process evaluation: Listening critically to other peoples' work

The following three tools developed by Jan Dewing, from various projects, can help you become a more effective active learner. They are useful for all team members. As you listen to your buddy or active learning group member or colleagues at meetings, you can use the prompts below to help you ask them questions. Some team members may need help to understand the prompts. If you do, ask someone who is involved in leading, coordinating or facilitating the development.

1. Hearing what is being said – **What does this mean to me and my work?**

2. Analysing what you hear from your point of view – **How does what I hear make sense to me (or not) from what I already know of the topic/issue?**

3. Exploring alternatives – **Am I aware of what alternatives I have not considered from what my buddy/ colleague has said?**

4. Considering the value of your understanding in the context of what you have heard – **How could my understanding help (through challenge and support) my buddy/colleague develop new insights?**

5. Helping my buddy/colleague make sense of the experience – **What questions can I ask my colleague to help them develop/clarify new/existing understandings?**

6. Being affirming – **How can I best demonstrate to my buddy/colleagues how I value them and what they have been talking about?**

Sheet 8.8: Process evaluation record: Listening skills

> Key question for reflection:
> How easy/difficult did I find what my buddy/active learning group members were presenting themselves and saying?

1. How easy/difficult did I find it to attend to what was said?
2. How easy/difficult did I find it to actively listen?   (Consider whether you kept your focus through everything that was said, how distracted you were and what these distractions were, and the level of sympathy/empathy you felt.)
3. How easy/difficult did I find it to attend to the person's non-verbal behaviour as they were talking?
4. How easy/difficult did I find it to keep a helpful distance from the person who was sharing?
5. How easy/difficult did I find interrupting the person's thoughts and feelings?
6. How easy/difficult did I find it to break a silence around what they were saying?
7. How easy/difficult did I find it to stay present throughout?
8. How easy/difficult did I find it to listen to the central content?
9. How easy/difficult was it for me to make value judgements and/or assumptions?

Sheet 8.9: Process evaluation record: What I said

Key question for reflection:
How easy/difficult did I find what I said?

1. What was the key focus of what I said?
2. What significant questions did I receive from my buddy/active learning group members?
3. What less helpful questions did I receive from my buddy/active learning group members?
4. What new Claims, Concerns or Issues did these questions raise for me?
5. What do I know now that I didn't know before?
6. What did I know that has now been reinforced for me?
7. What action do I need to take now?
8. What action do I want to take now?
9. How easy/difficult was it for me to be open and honest?
10. How easy/difficult was it for me to not say things and keep things back?

Sheet 8.10: Active learning evaluation

This evaluation form is suitable for all team members

1. Which two aspects of the session with your buddy/active learning group did you find most useful and why?

1)

2)

2. Which two aspects of the session did you find least useful and why?

1)

2)

3. What are the three most important aspects of learning for you today?

1)

2)

3)

4. What action(s) will you commit to as a result of today?

5. How effective were you in helping your buddy/active learning group members to learn for themselves?

6. How effective were they in enabling you to learn for yourself?

PART 3: Learning supervision

Part 3 is relevant to those people who have responsibility for providing learning supervision, for example registered nurses and therapists, managers and other clinical leaders. It is also useful for other team members who are interested in advancing their career through in-house and other educational opportunities.

Induction programmes, preceptorship, mentorship, coaching and work-based learning facilitation

Induction and preceptorship programmes

Induction or preceptorship programmes are offered to:

- promote the care of patients/residents and families;
- reduce the degree of stress people may experience as a new member of the team or going into a new role;
- ensure responsibilities are not placed on them too soon or inappropriately;
- minimise the risk to people, family members and themselves.

These programmes are tailored to the needs of the team and the kind of patients/residents and setting you work with and in, respectively. For example, a manager might work with a small team made up of a preceptor (person who supports the new staff member/person going into a new role) from each staff group to devise the programme. So whilst there are likely to be some core aspects of the programme that are relevant to all new staff who have no experience of working in care settings, such as working with older people, hygiene, fire regulations and the roles of the different staff groups, the design of the programme, kind of support given and the length of the programme will vary from a few weeks to several months according to the individual's learning needs.

The care manager and team might consider designing the programme around standards for the knowledge, skills and competencies for the various roles in the care setting. For example, the Social Care Institute for Excellence (SCIE) publishes on its website Common Induction Standards for adult social care, which could be used for care staff (http://search02.scie.org.uk/?q=Common%20Induction%20Standards).

In a good induction programme, each new team member receives support from an experienced team member (preceptor) to identify their learning needs, to develop a learning plan and to carry it out. For example, if some of the above standards were used in a programme, the preceptor might conduct relevant skills checks with an individual to help them develop their plan. Have a look at the examples of the Skills for Care / SCIE Skills Checks on the SCIE website (http://search02.scie.org.uk/?q=+Skills+Checks). The following topics might be relevant.

The organisation and role of the worker:

- person-centred support;
- effective communication;
- develop as a worker;
- principles of care;
- personal development.

The preceptor can draw on the resources in Part 2 of this chapter, especially the use of enabling questions to promote reflection, problem-solving and action planning. It can be helpful to draw up a list of enabling questions in advance and use the ones that then seem to fit best. They might also offer the new team member the opportunity to shadow them and watch what they are doing in the role. It is vital that the preceptor creates opportunities for the new team member to ask them questions about what they see, hear, feel and imagine, so that they can share their practical know-how and the knowledge that is usually so taken for granted that they don't think it is worth mentioning. And yet, for the new member in a team, it is vital.

For further information, by googling you can find a range of guidance materials that have been developed by the NHS in different areas of the country. You can search for these by googling NHS preceptorship. (www.nmc-uk.org/Documents/Circulars/2006circulars/NMC%20circular%2021_2006.pdf)

Supporting staff

Essential standards of quality and safety are set out by the Care Quality Commission. The Commission, now responsible for carrying out inspections of all registered health and social care settings, expects to see Regulation 23: Supporting workers in action:

Regulation 23: Supporting workers
People are kept safe, and their health and welfare needs are met, because staff are competent to carry out their work and are properly trained, supervised and appraised.

Many organisations take this responsibility seriously and offer training, learning, supervision and appraisal. Many of you will be very familiar with training opportunities like people and object moving and handling, food hygiene and risk assessment that your care setting provides or buys in for you from training services or colleges. Increasingly, the focus is more on learning rather than on training. Indeed training alone is insufficient to maintain improvements let alone innovation. In this chapter, we have shown how you can create person-centred learning culture and infrastructure and use active learning to enhance learning. Now we introduce you to learning supervision that can take several forms. You are probably already familiar with the first kind, that is, induction programmes. These programmes are designed to support you when you come into a new post or role in any care team or setting. You may also be familiar with the very similar preceptorship schemes that are offered in the NHS to support newly-qualified nurses over a 3–6 month period.

Once you have undertaken an induction or preceptorship programme and are gaining confidence in your practice, other learning supervision roles can be offered to enable continuous learning in the workplace. These include mentorship, coaching, and work-based learning supervision. Whilst these roles overlap in the helping styles and processes they use, they have different functions, which we show below.

Mentorship

Mentorship takes a longer term view and helps you to see the bigger picture of your career and what you would like to work towards. Your mentor is like a companion on your learning journey, offering you guidance and support in relation to your work. Mentors:

- help you reflect on your practice;
- help you learn through role-modelling and sharing the knowledge they have acquired through doing and learning on the job and any work-based learning they might have undertaken;
- offer you justified praise and celebrate in your achievements and successes – however small;
- give you feedback, as you have been learning to do in this workbook;
- ask you enabling questions to help you to discover your 'blindspots', analyse your issues and problems and work towards solutions and making good decisions;
- provide emotional and moral support;
- offer advice about your career, developing social contacts and building networks;
- introduce you to helpful contacts.

Coaching

Coaching focuses on helping you to improve some particular aspect of your practice. A coach helps you to draw on your own resources to improve the knowledge, know-how, skills and competencies you already have, rather than introducing you to new ones. A coaching style is thus recognised by collaborating, negotiating, involving and explaining processes.

The role of the coach is to help others to reveal to themselves the knowledge that is embedded in them and their practices that is invisible to them (and maybe others too). The coach helps them to bring it to the surface and to develop it further to bring about sustained learning and improvement. This is done mainly by asking enabling questions and high challenge/high support to help them to learn from their own resources. The coach will check that the person can successfully transfer their new learning to other situations. There may be times when the person is out of their depth, in other words has no inner resources or knowledge to draw on, and this is where it is necessary to switch to a more directing, mentoring style where the coach suggests ideas, structures the learning, shares what they know and guides the learner.

Work-based learning facilitation

Whilst everyday work in many care settings and homes is the basis for helping learning, development, evaluation and transformation in which all the above types of learning supervision can be used, work-based learning facilitation is more formal. This type of learning is generally facilitated by a partnership between an educational provider or a consultant and your organisation. You may have experienced work-based learning, if, for example, you have done a National Vocational Qualification or equivalent. It is likely that such learning will increase in the near future; for example, the foundation degree courses that are coming onstream will mean that work-based learning facilitators in care settings/

homes will be necessary. We therefore offer you, on the companion website, an example of what this might look like in an excerpt from a foundation degree guide developed by Claire Thurgate and colleagues. The guide is devised for people who have agreed to facilitate a colleague who has enrolled on a foundation degree within the Faculty of Health and Social Care at Canterbury Christ Church University.

Clinical or professional supervision for the future

If your team decides to set up the infrastructure for supervision of learning in the workplace, we suggest you look at the following website which has a huge resource of articles, papers and a video (www.supervisionandcoaching.com).

There are a number of PDF documents from different NHS organisations for different professional groups on the Internet. Just google *NHS clinical supervision* or *NHS policy on clinical supervision* to search for guidance that suits your needs. Or you could access and search your professional organisation's website.

Summary of learning in the workplace

By way of a summary of learning in the workplace, we offer Evans et al.'s (2006) advice on workplace learning.

- Remember that all workplaces are different. Tailor any interventions to the specifics of existing practices. Concentrate on what is feasible and possible, rather than idealistic goals.
- See analysing the learning culture as an important part of your job. This need not be either time consuming, or difficult. Take time to find out the answers to these important questions, through observation and informal conversations:
  - What are the barriers to learning in this workplace?
    - Can any of them be overcome?
    - Are there any valuable changes that can realistically be made?
    - What are the possibilities for learning here?
    - What valuable learning can be easily enhanced?
- Work with others. Most of the changes to a learning culture will lie beyond your direct influence. Can you help employers, middle managers, Trade Union leaders or groups of workers introduce valuable changes? Your presence in a workplace can be a valuable catalyst to the improvement of learning, partly through influencing the actions of others.

Finally, be realistic. In almost all workplaces, there will be important and desirable changes that, at the current time, are unachievable. Sometimes you have the best idea but the time isn't right so you need to revisit things at what becomes a better time. Meanwhile you can work on something else as there is always more development needed to work towards the vision and to maintain a person-centred workplace culture.

Useful websites

There are a lot of useful websites relevant to this chapter in addition to those presented in Chapter 1 of this workbook. As mentioned above, some of the resources are future oriented and perhaps a taste of what is to come. For ease of use, this section can also be accessed online (**www.wiley.com/go/practicedevelopment/workbook**).

1. **Campaign for Learning**
   This website is likely to be very useful for care setting managers generally in helping them to take the lead on creating a person-centred learning culture in the care setting. In particular, the *Leading on Learning: A hands-on guide for line managers* offers lots of ideas that match the values underpinning the person-centred learning we are promoting throughout this resource (www.campaignforlearning.org.uk/workplacelearningnetwork/ aboutworkplacelearning/resources_and_publications.asp).

2. **Care Quality Commission – Essential standards of quality and safety**
   These are the standards that are used by the Care Quality Commission to regulate adult social care providers. Regulation 23 is relevant here for supporting the need to develop the workforce in your social care setting:

   > **Regulation 23: Supporting workers**
   > People are kept safe, and their health and welfare needs are met, because team members are competent to carry out their work and are properly trained, supervised and appraised.

   (www.cqc.org.uk/)

3. **Social Care Institute for Excellence (SCIE)**
   Induction standards (revision recently launched) and related skills checks
   The Common Induction Standards were introduced in 2005. They were revised in June 2010. They are very relevant to learning in the workplace (see www.scie.org.uk/).
   In relation to these standards and in partnership with Skills for Care, SCIE has developed 8 Skills Checks that reference the 2010 common induction standards. Social care managers may find these skills checks very useful as they help team members to develop personal development plans. Each skills check includes the skills check activity, feedback form and personal development form. There is a huge range of skills check topics that can be easily accessed and downloaded.
   Regulation of health-care support workers (current thinking and exploration)
   To help you keep abreast of what is happening in relation to thinking about regulation of support workers in the health service, we have included this extract and these web pages.
   The Prime Minister's Commission recommends:

   > Some form of regulation of non-registered nursing and midwifery staff, including health care assistants and assistant practitioners, must be introduced to protect the public and ensure high quality care. The government and stakeholders must urgently scope and review options, and recommend what type and level of regulation are needed.

4. **Next steps**
   Health-care support workers (HCSWs) and their equivalents provide direct services related to patient care and treatment and support the work of registered nurses and midwives. There is currently no statutory provision for the regulation of HCSWs working in the UK.
   In January 2010, the Nursing and Midwifery Council (NMC) commissioned Professor Peter Griffiths and Dr Sarah Robinson of the National Nursing Research Unit at the Florence Nightingale School of Nursing and Midwifery based at King's College, London to analyse the risks and issues presented to public protection by unregulated HCSWs. (www.nmc-uk.org/Press-and-media/News-archive/Scoping-the-regulation-of-health-care -support-workers-/
   NMC clarifies its position on healthcare support workers (www.nmc-uk.org/Press-and-media/Latest-news/ NMC-clarifies-its-position-on-healthcare-support-workers/).
   This next document contains a report of the 'ongoing work being undertaken across the four United Kingdom countries and the Nursing & Midwifery Council (NMC) to explore the feasibility of healthcare support worker

(HCSW) regulation'. (www.nmc-uk.org/Documents/CouncilPapersAndDocuments/Committees/PPRC/22July2010/PPRC_10_16_RegulationOfHealthcareSupportWorkersUpdate.pdf)

You can keep up-to-date with this issue on the NMC website (www.nmc-uk.org),

where you can search for 'regulation of healthcare support workers'.

5. **National Vocational Qualifications (NVQs)**

This 'is a "competence-based" qualification: this means you learn practical, work-related tasks designed to help you develop the skills and knowledge to do a job effectively. NVQs are based on national standards for various occupations. The standards say what a competent person in a job could be expected to do. As you progress through the course, you compare your skills and knowledge with these standards as you learn, so you can see what you need to do to meet them. Taking an NVQ could be appropriate if you already have skills and want to improve them, or if you are starting from scratch'. (www.gov.uk/what-different-qualification-levels-mean)

You can browse the government website (www.gov.uk) and search for 'vocational qualifications' to find what you want to know. You can get information on the five different levels of NVQs, the entry requirements and how to find a course near you.

6. **Vocational qualifications on the Qualifications and Credit Framework (QCF)**

Vocational qualifications on the Qualifications and Credit Framework are new, work-related qualifications. They are designed to allow you to learn in a way that suits you, and give you the skills that employers are looking for. There are already lots to choose from, in a wide range of subjects.

(https://www.gov.uk/search?q=Vocational+qualifications+on+the+
Qualifications+and+Credit+Framework+)

7. **The NHS Knowledge and Skills Framework**

Although this framework was developed by the Department of Health for the NHS pay system and for developing post descriptions, it is also a framework that can be used to assess an individual's learning needs and plan how they will acquire the knowledge and skills that are required for their job. We include a brief description of the framework here because the dimensions of the framework are relevant to care home staff as well. It is worth looking at them for inspiration when you are thinking about your own personal development planning. (www.dh.gov.uk/en/Publicationsandstatistics/Publications/PublicationsPolicyAndGuidance/DH_4090843)

8. **Foundation Degrees**

Foundation degrees are higher education qualifications that integrate academic study with work-based learning. Designed jointly by employers, universities and colleges, they are available in a range of work-related subjects. (www.ucas.ac.uk/students/choosingcourses/choosingcourse/foundationdegree)

A foundation degree is equivalent to the first two years of an honours degree. It can be topped up by further study to an honours degree. The UCAS website above gives you more information about what is involved. These degrees are likely to replace the higher level NVQs in the future.

A demonstration foundation degree has recently been developed to enable care home staff to provide routine clinical patient care (www.skillsforhealth.org.uk/~/media/Resource-Library/PDF/Care_Home_Staff_Foundation_Degree.ashx).

Available from October 2010, the new qualification aims to offer relevant career progression and enable care home staff to enhance the comfort and treatment of residents within the care environment.

9. **Open University Foundation Degree in health and social care**

The Open University offers a one year Introduction to Health and Social Care course that provides an up-to-date, authoritative overview, with real-life case studies taking you deep into the experience of receiving care and working in care services. Whether you're involved in care work (paid or unpaid), use services yourself, or simply have a general interest, this course will help you to build knowledge and understanding, develop practical skills, and prepare for further study. (www3.open.ac.uk/study/undergraduate/course/k101.htm)

10. **Assistant Practitioners**

People working towards a foundation degree, may be interested in this new role that has been developed in the NHS and can equally apply in the care home sector.

Assistant practitioners work across a broad range of areas, mostly with direct service user contact. In the NHS, they will usually be managed by a healthcare professional, for example a dietician, nurse, occupational therapist, midwife, physiotherapist, operating department practitioner, or healthcare scientist.

Examples of assistant practitioner level roles include:

- occupational therapy assistant
- diabetes team assistant
- expert patient coordinator
- assistant theatre practitioner
- primary care worker in mental health
- dementia care worker
- IT support worker
- assistant practitioner (falls prevention).

(www.nhscareers.nhs.uk/details/Default.aspx?Id=2030)

11. **Competency frameworks or care pathways for care home and end-of-life staff**

   Another national trend developing is the use of competency frameworks or care pathways to improve the care a home can offer, for example the *End of Life Care Competencies* developed by St Christopher's Hospice (www .stchristophers.org.uk/competencies2012), the *NHS End of Life Care Pathway* (www.endoflifecareforadults.nhs.uk/ care-pathway) or *Principles in Palliative Care* developed by the Marie Curie Hospice (www.endoflifecareforadults .nhs.uk/).

12. **The Aged Care Channel: The TV Station for Care Homes**

   This member-driven training TV channel is available for all care home and nursing home staff on all shifts. The TV station broadcasts, via satellite, direct to your care home or nursing home so you can watch live and record a comprehensive schedule of programmes, covering all aspects of training. With leading practitioners demonstrating best practice, all programmes are filmed in real UK care homes. The subscription channel can be used for:

- delivering facilitated or self-directed learning;
- supporting a culture of continuous improvement;
- demonstrating current evidence-based practice;
- managing risk;
- promoting person-centred care;
- stimulating staff-empowerment;
- an annual programme of best practice programmes;
- live phone-ins to leading experts;
- integrated learning resources.

(www.agedcarechannel.co.uk/)

Chapter 9 What If . . .? When Things Don't Go So Well

Contents

Introduction

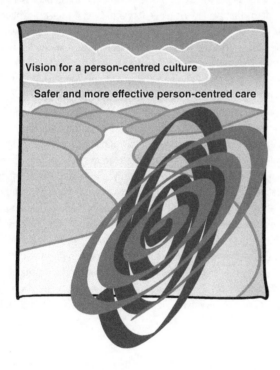

Vision for a person-centred culture

Safer and more effective person-centred care

Fig. 9.1 When things don't go so well

We are sure that you will have many successes and achievements on your practice development journey and this is why we have a bonus online chapter about sharing and celebrating on the companion website www.wiley.com/go/practicedevelopment/workbook. However, there are very likely to be times when things don't go as well as you might have expected or hoped for and you will need to be prepared for these occasions. Materials and activities in this chapter are for all members of the care setting team and stakeholders (those who have a stake in the thing not going so well).

Practice Development Workbook for Nursing, Health and Social Care Teams, First Edition. Jan Dewing, Brendan McCormack, and Angie Titchen.
© 2014 John Wiley & Sons, Ltd. Published 2014 by John Wiley & Sons, Ltd.
Companion website: www.wiley.com/go/practicedevelopment/workbook

Low spots are a reality of complex change. You should expect some low spots and prepare for them. Every practice development project has these times and we have been through it ourselves many times and seen others having similar experiences. However, there is hope – lots of it – and in this chapter we share with you how you can face up to and get around the most common challenges that many practice developers encounter as part of their work. Overcoming such challenges is what practice development is all about and many of the principles and processes we have introduced you to in this resource will help you navigate through tough times. The picture of our practice development path (Figure 9.1) gives you some clues. Do you notice how it is 'person-centred practice' and the spiral underneath the journey that are now the focus?

Working with challenges is best approached by being person-centred and using the processes you have been practising in this resource. We'll show you how to do this in this chapter.

When things don't go well, people often see this as 'going back to square one', 'going forward two steps and going back three' or 'falling down the snake in a game of snakes and ladders' – failing. We offer you the image of a spiral as another way of seeing things. The spiral represents our forward motion in that we learn through our mistakes. We learn about the bigger things going on inside the care setting and about the impact things outside, such as Government policy, have on the care setting, on you and on your organisation. Using this more energising symbol of the spiral, you reframe things not going well as an opportunity; a chance to learn, to problem-solve and figure out what stopped you achieving what you set out to. This can help you not to fall into the same trap again. Keep moving forward, learning and adapting rather than sitting still and doing too much analysis – this can cause paralysis.

Another energising idea to consider is that we always move forward. Even if it feels as though we have gone back, we can never do that because we, others and the situation have always changed in some way. When you go back to a place a second time it's never the same as the first time, just as we can never step into the same river twice (because the water is always flowing and changing). So, in this chapter, we try to show you that a crisis in the care setting or things going wrong can be reframed as an opportunity for learning and ongoing change.

A final word/picture – when you are trying to change things in the care setting and are then confronted with upheaval and difficulty, what has happened is like the unfreezing of a solid ice-cap (the ice-cap representing the care setting just going along doing things the way it always has done). When the ice is melting, it is much easier to change things before the next big freeze (the freeze representing the consolidation and sustaining of the changes you have brought about). So, the times when that might feel chaotic and unsettled are great times for practice developers to go about their work. What you need to do is make sure that you get the support you need to flow through the turbulence. Support will help you to deal with the negative emotions the turbulence might raise in you or the emotions of others that they try to push onto you. So here, we also offer you some guidance on how you might cope with troubled and icy waters.

Solution-focused thinking can help remind us that there are no problems, only opportunities. There is no failure, only learning. There is not just one solution (one truth), there are multiple solutions. There are no resistant, unmotivated, uncooperative people, only people with different ways of coping and cooperating.

As an estimate, try to spend 20% of your energy on analysing the problem and the remaining 80% on the solution. Focus the attention of others on the solution too. This doesn't mean you ignore or fail to develop an understanding of the problem. It means that you put most of your energy, individually and collectively, into finding solutions that will work for your care setting.

Resources in this chapter

- **Frequently asked questions** – to set the scene, we pose and answer the 'what if . . .' and 'How can I deal with . . .' questions that people ask at the beginning and throughout the practice development journey.
- **Most common challenges** – although each care setting and organisation and the people in it are unique, common challenges arise. We describe those challenges so that you can recognise them if they come up in your care setting. It often helps to know that others face similar problems. It also gives us hope to hear that other people have overcome them. We usually want to know how they did it, so we give you some examples so that you can learn from others' experiences.
- **Identifying why things are not going well** – sometimes things don't go well because we may have missed out a key step; for example, we may have excluded a key stakeholder and that person is blocking us from going forward or we may not have paid sufficient attention to including all stakeholders in the development of the vision statements. We present a checklist to help you hone in on any gaps/issues/problems/situations that might be the cause.
- **Material from other chapters of this resource that can be used for addressing the things that don't go well** – the table indicates material that you might find helpful for reframing, problem-solving and moving on when things seem impossible or you get upset or stuck.
- **Activities for helping you and others acknowledge what doesn't go well and efforts to learn, plan and change** – this sub-section builds on the activities in Chapter 8. Instead of focusing on achievements and successes, we help you to remember and honour them, and to focus on the negative and how to reframe it to move on.

Frequently asked questions

> Twenty-one questions that people frequently ask are set out below following the path of the practice development journey. The questions link with the most common challenges practice developers face. They are likely to be helpful to all team members and stakeholders as and when challenges present themselves.

When the possibility of doing practice development in your team or care setting is first discussed

Q1: How do we convince people that putting in all this effort will help improve the care experiences of patients/ residents and their families?

A1: You might consider the following:

- Sharing informally and formally, the experiences of other members of the care team and patients/residents who have improved not only the experience of being cared for in care settings, but also working and visiting in them. Formally, for example, you could show one of the videos pointed out in this resource in the website sections and have a discussion about it. Another idea is for a small group of you (including a resident if you work in a care home) to visit a care setting locally that has been developing and improving its practice and come back with photos and stories of what you have seen, felt and heard. You talk about those experiences in a staff meeting but also informally as you go about your work.

- Reading about the successes of other care settings in the sharing places of some of the websites mentioned at the end of the bonus online chapter (available at **www.wiley.com/go/practicedevelopment/workbook**) and having formal and informal discussions and conversations about these successes.
- Networking and/or visiting a care setting where they are working on similar projects and using practice development processes successfully.
- Identifying the full range of key stakeholders (Chapter 4) and getting them interested in the idea of practice development and its benefits for all patients/residents, families and team members.
- Talk with people who don't have a formal leadership role in the care setting but informally are very effective leaders of people – it is a good idea to get them on your side as early as possible.

Q2: How much is it going to cost? Where will the resources come from?

A2: Practice development can be done with no additional resources, providing staffing and skill-mix are adequate for people to take on new responsibilities. For some organisations it is helpful to have named staff with protected time to focus on getting practice development projects going. Becoming person-centred can, in the longer run, release staff time to engage in more learning activities and new or innovative care practices in the work place.

The main costs will be associated initially with freeing staff up to set up more effective structures and processes, to learn how to learn at work and help others to learn and to meet up to evaluate, plan, implement and evaluate the practice development plan. Costs for an external facilitator with practice development skills might be considered if there is no one in the setting with facilitation experience. As the aim for practice development is for it to become integrated as a way of life, once the initial investment has been made, practice development becomes absorbed into everyday work. Thus, costs are reduced as staff gain new skills and work more effectively and the workplace is run more efficiently. Cost-effectiveness studies are notoriously difficult to carry out because context and care are so complex, but increasing research is being done to test the effectiveness of practice development.

Funding for setting up a practice development initiative or the running of mini-projects within it could be sought from organisations that support innovation and improvement, for example The Foundation of Nursing Studies (www.fons.org/), or you could check out whether your organisation holds development funds that could be applied for. Finding someone in your organisation who would be supportive and could help you access charitable funds or small amounts of funding can also help. Think about people in Clinical Governance, Learning and Development or in Workforce Development roles.

A business plan will be necessary for larger scale practice development projects and this would be put together by the care setting manager and other senior managers in the organisation. Plans should make use of national policy themes and targets. For example, using the Department of Health's National Dementia Strategy as the starting point, a business plan would demonstrate how the care setting needs to invest in its workforce to enable them to improve the care of patients/residents with dementia.

The business plan could be informed and justified by data from the early stages of the baseline evaluation.

Q3:   How can we take on more work when we are already over-stretched?

A3:   At the beginning, this question is probably the most asked. Practice development is commonly seen as more or extra work on top of existing work. At this stage, it is rare that people see practice development as necessary for doing their jobs more efficiently and effectively. In addition, the setting may not have a learning culture, so learning in and from work is not done. Rather, learning is seen as separate from and on top of existing work. As a learning culture develops, people's attitudes change as they experience the benefits of doing practice development and learning and they find that they can usually make time. Moreover, based on evaluation evidence, some work practices might be dropped and other more efficient and effective ways are developed which save time (see next sub-section for more ideas). It's important to ask team members to see what they can do: so using questions such as 'what can you do?' and 'what are you prepared to do?' can help focus.

Q4:   Why should I be involved? Surely it is management that should be doing this? Or what if I didn't get involved?

A4:   It's vital to stress and keep restressing: everyone is being asked to become involved including managers. However, this approach won't work and can't be as successful as it might without all the team making a contribution.

You may feel able to say it is expected that everyone will demonstrate their support. You should say clearly what this will look like in terms of behaviours.

There have been many studies that show that collaborative change approaches that involve everyone's commitment and participation at all levels of the organisation, to different degrees and in different ways, are more effective and sustained in the longer term than top-down approaches. So if you don't take up the opportunity to participate, then the development of person-centred practices is likely to be severely limited.

Q5:   What if no one except very few staff and patients/residents want to do or are actively resisting the practice development? What do we do then?

A5:   An effective way of working in both these situations is to work with the few staff and patients/residents who are keen to get involved. Very quickly, stakeholder engagement and communication plans should be developed and implemented by this small group. As staff and patients/residents who were uninterested or resistant begin to hear about what is going on and notice the differences the practice development is making in terms of benefits for them, more people will begin to commit. You are likely to find that you get a snowball effect as more and more people join in.

At the same time you should also work with these people to see what it is they want to see happen or to understand more about their reasons for not wanting change. A person's identity may be closely bound with the problem or an existing way of doing things. By externalising 'the problem' we create 'space' between the problem and the person – the cracks that can let the light in.

Q6:   What's in this for me? Why should I be bothered?

A6:   Being involved in practice development brings benefits to patients/residents, families and members of the care team (see Chapters 6 & 7 for examples you can refer to and consider). For patients/residents and families, they begin to feel listened to and treated as a unique person. They get to know who is looking after them better and vice versa. The result is person-centred relationships that are more deeply satisfying and life enhancing for those within them. As team members get to know the patient/resident and family members, they are better able to provide care and services that are uniquely tailored to the needs of patients/residents and family members. Such care provision is more satisfying than care given in routine, unthinking and in de-personalising ways. In addition, team members' careers may benefit from learning in the workplace and developing practice development skills that are transferable to other contexts. Enhanced knowledge and skills may lead to career advancement.

It may seem to you from the answer above (and from what you may have seen as you browsed through the resources and activities) that practice development is really only for care settings where patients are there for a long period of time or where those needing care are older, severely cognitively impaired or are residents in a long-term rehabilitation setting or care home. We want to stress really strongly that the journey to a person-centred culture through practice development is as highly relevant to acute, short-term care settings as to long-term care. You only have to pick up a newspaper, watch the TV news or have been an in-patient yourself to be aware that care in many kinds of acute health settings is far from person-centred. So whether you work in an acute setting like a critical care unit, a short-term setting like a clinic or day-case ward, or a long-term setting like a nursing home, the principles, processes and outcomes of practice development are equally relevant to you. The principles guide you in modifying the stakeholder engagement and the processes you use and in how you use them in your particular setting. For example, if you work in a day-case ward, you could engage patients in a Claims, Concerns and Issues activity at their follow-up out-patient visits or you could invite former patients to gather other patients' stories as they wait in the out-patient clinic.

When you start working on developing a shared vision for person-centred care

Q7:   *Some of us contributed to the values clarification activity, but many staff members were not on duty that day and a lot of patients/residents were not there either. How can we make sure that they have the chance to contribute to the values clarification? What if we can't get everyone to contribute? What do we do then?*

A7:   Having difficulty in getting everyone involved is a very common situation. You could think about doing the activity over three weeks so that it gives many more people the opportunity to join in. There is a guide on how to do this in Chapter 3. If some people still don't contribute, then the offer for them to be included at any time, in their own way, is made widely known. Any approaches for late inclusion are warmly welcomed and followed up as soon as possible. No blame is attached for late or no contributions. Values and beliefs work should always be revisited, so make sure people know when that opportunity will arise.

Q8:   *Having got some people onboard, how can we carry their involvement through to the vision statement workshop we are planning?*

A8:   Getting stakeholder commitment through engaging with a Claims, Concerns and Issues activity, for example, and developing a stakeholder communication plan are vital for ensuring that everyone knows about and is committed to developing a shared vision (see Chapter 4).

When you are getting started on measuring and evaluating

Q9:   *Who should carry out the measuring and evaluating?*

A9:   The idea that all stakeholders can be involved in all aspects of practice development should be promoted right at the beginning of the journey. However, others need to know that time frames do apply as work needs to progress. Therefore, it shouldn't come as a surprise that many of the stakeholders have the opportunity to carry out the measuring and evaluation with the support of the practice development coordinating group (see Question 14) and that feedback will be offered to all stakeholders

Q: 10   *What if we don't get the commitment of many stakeholders to do the baseline evaluation, what do we do so that we can develop a practice development plan based on evidence?*

A10:   As in our answer to Question 5, start with those stakeholders who show interest. Their enthusiasm and energy will draw others in when they see the benefits. Ask yourself whether you are collecting the sort of evidence that the stakeholders value – it may be that compromise is needed or that you need to convince some stakeholders further.

Q11:   *How can we involve stakeholders in gathering the evidence when everyone is so busy and the care team members work shifts?*

A11:   The answer parallels our response to Question 3 above. As the culture begins to shift towards a learning culture and a culture of effectiveness, team members become more adept and empowered at managing their time efficiently and making work priorities in order to make time for gathering evidence and supporting others who want to contribute. In addition, patients/residents and family members might choose to contribute, which shares the workload, as well as promoting genuine collaboration, inclusion and participation of stakeholders. Shift working may not be a hindrance because evidence can be collected across a 24 hour time span in many cases. Indeed, if there is an overlap of those shifts, there are more team members on duty and this is an ideal time to gather evidence.

Q12:   *I am not qualified to do evaluation, so if I am asked to participate, what do I do?*

A12:   You do not need to be a registered health-care professional to be involved. It's most important that you want to learn and are open to learning including feedback. If you are not offered support when you are asked to participate it would be good for you to ask for detail about what you are being invited to do, that is, which method of gathering evidence would you be expected to use and what support you could be offered. When you have narrowed it down, you could read about the method, say for example, patient/resident/relative narrative interviews in Chapter 5 of this workbook. As you read, make notes of things you don't understand and questions you want to ask before you commit to helping. It is also important to say what support you need to contribute before you commit. Remember you might surprise yourself if you have a go.

When you get going on developing the practice development plan

Q13:   *Who should analyse the baseline evidence? Who should develop and carry out the plan? If I am to be involved, how do I prepare myself?*

A13:   As in response to Question 9, any stakeholder can be involved in the analysis of evaluation evidence and the development of the plan. If you are interested in participating, look on the noticeboards in the care setting to find out who the contact person is or ask the practice development coordinating group (if you have one) or manager. You can prepare yourself by discussing with them, what it will involve and by looking at Chapters 5 & 6 and making notes of what you don't understand or want more information on, the questions you want to ask and the support you will need before you commit to helping. The best preparation is to imagine what the evidence might say and how you might feel about things you hear that aren't as positive as you might like. Being open to feedback and to listening is vital.

Q14: How can we develop the plan efficiently and cost-effectively?
A14:   You may find that the most efficient and cost-effective way, in terms of reducing duplication of effort, is to set up a practice development coordinating group of key stakeholders (Chapter 4). It is good to recruit members from across the whole team, patients/residents and family members. This group would be responsible for setting up systematic structures and processes to ensure efficient planning and communication. Developing plans should be made available for stakeholders to comment on if they wish, perhaps using a Claims, Concerns and Issues activity. This open approach whilst it may seem time-consuming, results in a plan that is owned and to which people are prepared to commit because their ideas and views have been listened and responded to.

Q15: What can we do if we discover that we have been unrealistic about what we can achieve?
A15:   You could go back to your practice development plan, check that you have used the overview action planning template and use the SMART/SMARTER guidelines to ensure that this time your goals are Specific, Measurable, Agreed upon, Realistic, Time-based, Energising and Recorded. Then you can do a self-assessment of the revised plan and send it out for review by stakeholders. You ask them to consider how realistic the goals are now with the changes that have been made. Supporting materials are in Chapter 6.

When our mini-projects are underway

Q16: We already have two mini-projects going and a small group of care staff are keen to start another one. I am worried though. My question is 'Are we in danger of over-burdening these patients/residents (some of whom are frail) what with all the evidence we are supposed to collect to develop and evaluate our mini-project plan?'
A16:   This is a really good question because it is very important not to over-burden patients/residents and team members with the task of providing evidence (to ensure a sound and realistic plan and then to evaluate the impact of the project on peoples' experiences). When you have several projects already going, it may be possible to look at and use evidence that has already been collected by another project or it may be possible to 'piggy-back' future evaluations by another project group or plan one together to avoid duplication. This is where having a practice development coordinating group is a good idea because they can keep the various project groups up-to-date with where each other is at and whether there is a possibility for doubling up on collecting information or taking action.

When learning in the workplace gets underway (which should be all the way along the practice development journey!)

Q17: How can I find the learning support I need in my care setting when there are no systems or processes in place to help me get it?
A17:   If you haven't already, you could find yourself a buddy and work together on the activities in this resource. You could also approach your manager or team leader, as they are likely to be responsible for work-based learning in your setting, to discuss putting a system and processes in place so that staff can continue to learn and improve their practice. You could even offer to help, for example, to set up a register of people who already have experience of helping others to learn. You could do this in a variety of ways, by talking to your co-workers to find out if any of them have experience of being a preceptor, mentor, coach or supervisor or by putting a notice up on the staff board or in the care setting newsletter. Even if only one person responds, it is a start. Building on the information you have collected and presented to your manager or team leader, they might invite you and this one person to join them in a task group with the purpose of developing learning support for staff. At the beginning, this might mean buying in a facilitator to train a group of interested staff to become learning helpers. As they gain experience through using the activities in this resource, they begin to help other staff members to develop their helping skills. In this way, the register of people able to offer help gets bigger. See also Chapter 8 for identifying and finding the learning support you need.

Q18: I have tried to give my co-workers feedback when things go wrong, using the ideas in this resource, but I meet resistance every time. What should I do?
A18:   Three golden principles to use whenever things don't go well are (1) to return to the vision statement, (2) to revisit the ground rules you have developed with these co-workers and (3) don't start with negative feedback. These principles are three fundamental things that these people will have signed up to (if practice development based on the

Collaboration, Inclusion and Participation principles has been adhered to). Check to see whether the vision statement includes anything about the care setting working towards a learning culture. If it does, you can discuss with these co-workers what they and you think a learning culture is. You might say that giving and receiving feedback non-defensively is vital if we are to learn from our work. What do your ground rules say about this? If there is nothing about receiving feedback non-defensively, you could negotiate it in. Another thing to check out, using the materials about feedback in this resource (Chapters 5 & 8), is whether you gave the feedback in a challenging, *yet supportive way*. Why not negotiate to practise giving feedback with your buddy and get his or her feedback on how it made her or him feel and how helpful or not it was. Finally, ask the team members how they would like feedback offered to them.

Q19:   *Although there is lip service to learning at work being important in the workplace, when I have tried, repeatedly, to negotiate 15 minutes to reflect on something in the shift overlap, whoever is in charge that day always says 'There isn't time – you'll have to do it at home'. With a young family, this is not possible for me. I want to learn, so what should I do?*

A19:   The first thing to do is to think a bit more about what the reasons are for the responses you get. For example, do you relate your request to a specific resident or provide a rationale that will mean something to others? Look at these two examples and decide which would get most support?

'I want 15 minutes to reflect please.'

'I want to take 15 minutes to think about the way Mrs Lang's behaviour has changed recently and how we can better respond to it. I will update the care plan.'

You might want to choose an opportunity carefully where you can raise the issue with your co-workers and ask them about their reasons. If there is a Claims, Concerns and Issues activity going on (or you arrange one), then you could raise your experiences. Be careful to raise your concern or issue in a sympathetic way that attaches no blame to anyone and does not assume your solution. Rather you point out the mismatch and then turn your concern into the issue (question): 'How can we ensure we are learning in the workplace within the time we have available to us?' When you get to discussing this question with your co-workers in a team meeting, for instance, you might conclude that people say there is no time because that is what we always say, even if we could make time by prioritising our work or helping each other out with the work to give the other 15–20 minutes with their learning buddy. Then next time, it is vice versa.

When it's time to share and celebrate

Q20:   *We've been very good at sharing and celebrating our successes in the unit/ward/home along the way, but now we are so proud of what we have achieved we feel that we need to share our successes in the community or even nationally so that others can benefit! The thought terrifies us, so how can we do this and prepare ourselves for such a challenge?*

A20:   If you have been sharing your successes along the way, you have been developing the skills you need for sharing outside the setting! These are your communication and presentation skills. You can prepare yourself by doing a bit of reading about how to communicate and present ideas in public. There are loads of books on this and your local library is bound to have one or two, or you could browse the Internet for tips. But by far the best way is to rehearse your communication or presentation with your buddy, co-workers and patients/residents and get feedback from them about what went well and what could be improved. The important things are to take a few deep, relaxing breaths before you begin, tell yourself that you can do it, focus on the people who are there being able to hear what you have to say and then be yourself as you share your achievements and successes.

When it's time to keep it fresh

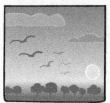

Q21:   *How can we sustain our enthusiasm for practice development as a way of being, living and working? What if we get tired and lose our enthusiasm?*

A21: It is important to recognise that there may be times when new things become embedded and part of the way we do things around here, that we might lose our motivation for continually improving things. We get comfortable again. That is only natural. To sustain our enthusiasm for the long haul, we can think of practice development as a flock of geese migrating. Sometimes, we are leading the way, sometimes we are supporting others to lead and then we take our turn again. We do need to pace ourselves, especially as the energy and excitement that doing practice development brings can cause us to overdo it. So we need to be mindful that this can happen and take steps to nurture ourselves for the next steps on the journey which, for example, might be about keeping our new practices fresh through evaluation or linking them to new policy agendas (see the bonus online chapter at **www.wiley.com/go/ practicedevelopment/workbook**).

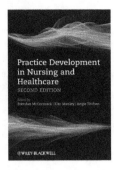

And remember, McCormack et al. (2013) can also be a resource to help you think through how to respond to the challenges you encounter. This more theoretical book contains up-to-date thinking on practice development that is illustrated with real-life examples of practice development including some of the aspects that don't go according to plan.

Most common challenges

> Common challenges that people face in doing practice development and being and becoming practice developers are reflected in the Questions and Answers above. These challenges occur in many different types of health and social care settings and care homes. Here we show how these challenges play out and how others have overcome them.

1. Heavy workloads

Perceived heavy workloads are almost always the biggest challenge to overcome. Developing effective staff–patient/resident/family member relationships require having enough time to spend with patients/residents without a constant feeling of being 'rushed'. It is common for this feeling to arise from, and be driven by, a routinised and task-oriented culture. Often practitioners themselves play a large part in creating and sustaining this culture and do not recognise their role in this.

> However, through practice development activities such as structured reflection and observations of practice, staff can be helped to explore for themselves the effectiveness of teamwork, workload management, time management and staff relationships and make changes that enable more effective management of workload. For example, in the Irish practice development programme (McCormack et al., 2010) featured in this resource, staff engagement in such activities contributed to an altered perspective and a desire to act on this. With collective action, this contributed to a change in culture where there was a greater sense of 'helpfulness' in teamwork. Data collected in reflective journals maintained by participants and observation of practice records reinforced this finding, such as:
>
> > We have been overly obsessed by tasks in my unit and I am developing a greater awareness of how this gets in the way of being person-centred. However, it is only when we all develop a similar awareness that we can become truly person-centred in the way we work
> >
> > (Participant's reflective note)
>
> Team members started the day by reviewing how they would schedule the different activities that needed to be done with patients/residents and identified who needed to be involved. The plan included those activities (such as showering) that could be undertaken in the afternoon as a more 'therapeutic activity' as opposed to a 'morning task' . . . it was good to see team members check with each other what help they needed with their work. (Time 2 observation note)

2. Working in care settings with older people (especially those with dementia) is hard work

If the staff are exposed to 'impoverished' environments of care in which poor standards of care and negative attitudes towards older people dominate, many team members are likely to have negative predispositions towards older people. This leads to staff experiencing their work as hard and older people as 'difficult' and 'demanding'. However, if 'enriched' environments are experienced, this is likely to encourage positive attitudes towards older people and their care, which leads to reduced perceptions of stress and increased satisfaction in the workplace.

> Thus it is important to focus on changing workplace culture in health care and residential care environments and maximise the opportunities available for care staff to engage in person-centred relationships with colleagues, patients/residents, families and communities.

3. Doing practice development in times of major financial pressure and economic cut-backs

Times are hard right now for developing practice and cutbacks in external education and travel are likely.

> If learning is enabled to happen in the care setting itself, then developments will continue. Additionally, staff are more likely to have a greater intention to stay in the work setting. This is demonstrated in the international literature that shows the importance placed on access to education and learning and that this access combined with available opportunities for career advancement are more important than 'pay' in itself. Learning vitality contributes to thriving in the workplace. In addition, thriving promotes resilience, flourishing and more positive self-evaluations. Creating the conditions for learning through active learning, as presented in this resource, brings about willingness of staff and patients/residents to think of new ideas, explore new possibilities and behave creatively.
>
> Developments in the workplace culture are likely to enable staff to make better use of the staff complement and to develop more effective ways of working together. This suggests a shift in the practice culture to one where staff support each other better, make better use of their resources and which engages them more in effective collaborative working.
>
> Consider putting forward a case for using the time released for care from projects in The Productive Series[1] to undertake new activities such as carrying out observations of care and gathering patient stories.

4. Lack of management support

The involvement of managers in practice development is crucial to the successful implementation of practice development processes and the sustainability of outcomes. Lack of support can be devastating and even undermining as shown in one of the residential care settings in the Irish study (McCormack et al., 2010):

> . . . The work was so unsupported and undermined that at times it was difficult to know how it could continue. The challenges she [internal facilitator] faced were so non-person-centred and critical that it fuelled the staff who were resistant to change. This meant that every little development was hugely challenging and was continually undermined.

In contrast, supportive management leads to success and the achievement of practice development plans:

> Ongoing support from management was crucial to the success of the [practice development], facilitating the release of participants and supporting the ongoing action plans proved vital in the current cost containment environment. Management's acknowledgement of the need for the [practice development] and seeing it as a vital link in maintaining standards also helped me work effectively.
>
> (Internal Facilitator's Reflection)

Practice development focuses on empowering staff to develop skills that enable them to make changes themselves, to do so in a critical and reflective way and to learn how to use those skills repeatedly in their practice. Without the support of managers, such growth, development and self-exposure falls on barren ground, is limited when the interface with management is encroached and the benefits are never fully realised. Here's what happened in the Irish practice development programme:

> A wonderful programme for team building and getting all grades working together for the benefit of the [patients/residents] – changing the culture and involving [patients/residents] in their daily care and giving choice to patients/residents, thus empowering them and improving staff morale. The role of the Internal Facilitator has been critical. Strong leadership is required to bring all staff onboard with person-centredness and reflective practice – a must to learn from actions. Continuous feedback to all stakeholders is so important . . .
>
> (Reflection from Director of Nursing)

---

[1] **The Productive Series** focuses on improving processes and environments to help nurses and therapists spend more time on patient care, thereby improving safety and efficiency.

Whilst effective practice development can take place in spite of a lack of support by the manager, it is greatly eased if the manager is supportive. So if it is a group of staff or senior managers who decide they want to use this resource to develop person-centred care, then it is a good idea to get the support of the manager right at the beginning.

> In summary, adequate staffing levels, good inter-professional relationships and effective management/leadership in the care setting, (requisites of person-centred practice), have causal links with higher levels of professional satisfaction and care workers' ability to engage in person-centred practice with patients/residents. Participants in the Irish programme were seen to shift their orientation of caring from one where technical tasks were given greater priority to one where relationships with patients/residents and families were more highly valued. This finding (the first in residential care settings) supports other international research in health care which suggests that there is a direct relationship between the attributes of an effective workplace culture and patient outcomes.

5. Making practice changes is not easy

We cannot pretend that developing person-centred practice will be easy. It isn't, because it challenges individuals, teams and organisations at the core level of values and beliefs. Sometimes when a new team member begins working in a care setting, they might notice that certain practices or ways of doing things in the care setting are not person-centred or even bordering on the abusive, but after a period of time, they too become so familiar with this way of working, they no longer see it. It is really hard to overcome routinised, habitual ways of working, and the only way individuals, teams and organisations can do it is to become aware and stay aware through learning.

The essence of the practice development approach we have used in this resource is that of changing 'self' (i.e. adjusting my perspective(s) of situations and then acting accordingly). This requires considerable commitment and dedication of staff to engage in the analysis of 'self'. The discomfort and crises that occur when routines and behaviours are challenged requires skilled facilitation. These facilitation interventions are not a one-off event but re-occur to form a pattern until the individual can transcend the routinised practice.

A frequent crisis is when people become aware that whilst espousing one set of values and beliefs (e.g. saying openly that they share the values and beliefs that make up the vision statement for person-centred care), they then realise, often with a shock, that they are actually living another set (e.g. giving care that is centred on the needs of the care setting and not on the patients/residents' needs). Without skilled facilitation, some people remain unaware of such paradoxes as they go about their everyday work. Helping people to recognise this mismatch in their own practice is challenging for facilitators. It is also challenging for them to engage care team members who feel threatened by such approaches. It is difficult for facilitators to 'hold' these team members as they make their journeys in coming to terms with the realities of practice and to maintain momentum so that real changes can occur within a set time frame.

> It is vital that care settings support team members in developing their facilitation skills. The learning activities in this resource have been designed to help all care team members to do that. However, the development of person-centred practice will be more effective if a care setting employs someone with facilitation skills. For example, if a care setting requires nursing staff, then it could look for these skills when appointing these staff. Or a group of care settings could consider employing a skilled facilitator in this practice development approach to support staff in developing their practice to meet requirements for person-centred care. Better still, this skilled facilitator could act as a mentor or coach to help an internal facilitator in each care setting to develop their skills and support them in their work. In addition, bringing internal facilitators together would not only increase their opportunities for learning support, it would also provide networking opportunities for sharing achievements and successes in changing practice.

6. Scepticism about patients/residents being able to contribute to practice development

Another challenge is care team members being sceptical about asking patients/residents about their experiences. In addition, the frailer and more cognitively impaired the person is, the less likely it is that staff will believe that this person had anything to offer in terms of knowledge. In the Irish practice development programme, life experiences were regarded as stories that may or may not be truthful. Connected to this there was a high level of concern about whether what patients/residents said was truthful or not. Through a range of programme activities and the narrative evaluation method, participants were able to come to value that truth is not fixed and not even the priority when it comes to life stories, narratives and reminiscences. At the beginning, the teams were genuinely surprised that patients/residents experienced a reluctance to be open and honest about their views on care. Maybe this was because they passively accepted that the care setting team would know best.

> I thought that we knew best what was good for the [residents]. Now I know that we don't and even if we do, it's not always what the [resident] wants. This programme has shown me that what I know is important but how I talk to and value what they [residents] want and do not want is more important.
>
> (Participant's reflection year 2)

Patient/resident committees can be set up to provide structures through which patients/residents can have a voice in how services are provided. It is well documented that these forums can take a long time to become effective. They require skilled facilitation to ensure that the patients/residents are genuinely voicing their views and that these views are representative of all patients/residents. Evidence that this is possible is that across the Irish sites, residents' committees were consulted on a range of issues such as name badges, mealtimes and menu choices, special events (parties), decor, furnishings and pets.

Another challenge is promoting staff learning alongside patients/residents. In this resource, we have offered you ideas and activities for enabling shared learning to occur.

> There is universal acceptance of the need for patient/resident involvement (or engagement) in practice development work. Making this happen will involve the care team going through a process of learning how to learn from and with those they care for.

7. Initial difficulty in working with the principles of Collaboration, Inclusion and Participation (CIP)

Throughout this resource, we have promoted the importance of the key principles of collaboration, inclusion and participation (CIP) when working with stakeholders. Whilst you may try out the activities we have suggested in this resource to identify and engage them, you may sometimes encounter initial disinterest or resistance. If you do, here are some things you can try.

- Help people to see that practice development is:
  - a long-term investment;
  - everybody's business;
  - a way of life and work, through which everyone benefits;
  - self-sustaining and thereby cost-effective;

  and that it is not:
  - a top-down, quick fix.
- Try to convince people, especially managers, leaders and executives that although quick, slick fixes (that usually have acronyms and glossy materials) may be attractive in the short term, their track record suggests that they often don't have a lasting effect on practice and the context and culture of the organisation or service. Can you think of any quick fixes in the past in your area that failed to bring about sustained changes and which you can refer to when you are trying to convince these people?

- Show them the benefits of practice development by drawing on the examples in the bonus online chapter at **www.wiley.com/go/practicedevelopment/workbook**

Example

A few months ago, the executive board of an acute care Trust discussed the implications of the National Dementia Strategy document put out by the Department of Health. They know that they need to be seen to be doing something about developing the workforce, so that the Trust provides person-centred dementia care to patients. They have decided that they have to make this investment and have agreed to buy in the services of a training company to come and do some mandatory sessions on dementia for all staff.

Meanwhile, service managers have responded favourably to the board about their intention to invest in staff development. They explain that they would like to take the opportunity to put forward a proposal to the board to introduce practice development into the Trust, based on the experience of staff in the medical unit who have demonstrated improvements in the care of patients with strokes. The proposal, created by the care staff and patients, taps into the National Dementia Strategy. It shows how practice development will be a cost-effective, long-term investment for the Trust and could result in the Trust becoming a centre of excellence just as the demographic time bomb is going off. By this they mean that there will be many more people with dementia needing to be cared for. The proposal points out that research has shown how one-off training sessions have little or no long-term impact on changing practice. The board are impressed and invite the service manager and representatives of the staff and patients to come along to the next board meeting to tell them more about what practice development is and how it works.

Identifying why things are not going well

> This 'checklist' might be helpful to those leading, coordinating and facilitating the development of practice in exploring the cause of things that are not going well. Team members may also find the checklist useful. The table that follows points out the material in this resource that you can then use to start putting things right.

Checklist

- **Revisiting your vision statement** – a good starting point for when things are not going so well is to revisit your vision statement.
- **Using personal reflection tools** (available on the companion website) **and creative visualisation activity** – if you have been directly involved in something that did not go well, using a personal reflection tool might help you to identify that this was because of something that you did or didn't do or be. In this case, using a reflection tool could help you to unpick what you did and what happened so that you can learn from it and develop action points for moving on.
- **Reflecting with a helper** – often we need help to reflect upon our own experience. By using a reflective tool to prepare for a reflection session with a helper (who might be your buddy or team leader, for example) or your preceptor/mentor/clinical supervisor if you have one, reflecting with someone else can help you to go further in your understanding and therefore action planning. For instance, your buddy/preceptor/mentor/clinical supervisor may help you, through enabling questions, to recognise blindspots that your reflection alone didn't bring up. When you become aware of them, then you can plan what you will do about it. The person helping you might also give constructive feedback and give you emotional support if you need it.
- **Doing a Claims, Concerns and Issues activity** – if the thing that didn't go well involves others, then it is important to remember the Collaboration, Inclusion and Participation (CIP) principles. To get the ball rolling, doing this activity with relevant stakeholders helps you to clarify the issues (questions) that you, as a group, need to attend to and develop an action plan for.
- **Using the problem-solving tool** (available on the companion website) – if you as an individual or a group of stakeholders know there is a problem to be addressed, this tool can help you or the group to analyse the problem to better understand it. Action planning can then be better informed. The tool helps you to keep track of the action and its effect.
- **Being solution focused** – using solution focused questions can help new options and possibilities to emerge. Here are some examples of solution focused questions:
  - On a scale of 0–10, where 10 equals us at our very best, where are we now?
  - What have you/we done well so far to get to there?
  - What needs to happen for you/us to go on progressing up the scale?
  - What will you/we be doing differently at the next step up? How will you (or stakeholders) be able to tell?
  - Let's suppose that you/we get to the next step up tomorrow. What's the smallest sign that will tell you that things are improving?
    - What else will you/we see?
    - And what else . . .?

Sheet 9.1: Material from other chapters in this resource that can be used for addressing things that don't go well

Chapter	Material	How you could use the material
Chapter 1	Practice development framework	Look at the framework to see whether you and the care setting are attending to all the elements of the framework. Identify which part of the framework you need to pay attention to to resolve the particular issue you are working on.
	Practice development principles	Relate the principles to your current situation. How can you put the principles into practice in the action plan you develop to move through this difficulty?
	Person-centred practice framework	Which of the four parts of the framework do you need to pay attention to? • *prerequisites*, which are the qualities and skills of staff in the care setting • *the care environment*, which focuses on the setting in which care is delivered • *person-centred processes*, which focus on delivering care through a range of activities • *expected outcomes*, which are the results of effective person-centred practice
Chapter 2	Reflection on my own values and beliefs	Looking back over the work you did at the beginning of the practice development journey (in your learning notebook if you kept one when you did this activity originally), reflect now on whether your own values and beliefs reflect those in the vision statement of the care setting that you all created together. If they don't, you could reflect with your buddy/preceptor/mentor/clinical supervisor why they don't and what you could do.
	Going for a reflective walk on your own or with your learning buddy	You could redo this reflective walk on your own or with your buddy to compare what you found out then about the hidden values in the care setting and whether you now see any changes as a result of you all trying to live the values of the vision statement. If you don't, reflect on why you see no differences.
	Values and beliefs of the care setting	You might want to look back at the notes you made with your buddy as you walked around your care setting as if you were a patient or potential resident. Would you feel the same now if you walked around the care setting again? Are there any differences? Are there any clues here about why the thing you are concerned with didn't go well?
	Leaders' values and beliefs	If you are a leader in the care setting, look at the notes you made if you did this activity. Are your values reflected in the new vision for the care setting? Are you living the values you expressed there and those in the vision statement? Does a mismatch of values account for what is not going well?
	Worksheet for recording learning activities with a buddy: Values and beliefs about care	Check out what you have been writing on your worksheet. Are there any mismatches with your values and what is happening in relation to the things that are not going well?
Chapter 3	Visualisation through painting and/or collage (workshop guidance)	A way to start thinking about how you can address the things that are not going well is to visualise the outcome you want to achieve and how you might get there. You could do it through visualisation in a way similar to what you may have done when you were developing the shared vision for your care setting. You can use the same ideas to work on your own or with others, perhaps in a meeting set up to address the issue.
	Visioning (workshop guidance)	The same goes, as just above, for the processes in this workshop guidance.
Chapter 4	Reflection tools (available on companion website)	You can use these tools for reflecting on yourself in relation to what didn't go well (as well as what did go well). For example, in negotiating time to carry out a values clarification activity, engaging key stakeholders, helping someone else to learn, facilitating a meeting, carrying out your part of the practice development plan or in a situation where you did not live person-centred values.
	Getting the commitment of stakeholders A template for stakeholder views: Claims, concerns and issues Guidance on facilitating Claims, concerns and issues	It is important for all key stakeholders to participate in tackling what is not going as planned or unexpected problems or difficulties that arise during the action.
Chapter 5	SWOT or TOWS tool	This tool can be useful in assessing in this new situation what you can build on (strengths and opportunities) and what you need to do some work on (weaknesses and threats).
Chapter 6	Overview action planning guide Overview action planning template (available on companion website)	You might want to revisit this planning guide and template if you need to develop new action plans to address what hasn't gone according to plan.

Chapter	Material	How you could use the material
	Action point planning sheet (available on companion website)	We point this sheet out here as a reminder that it is important to record action points – sometimes things don't go well because we might have forgotten what we agreed to do!
	SMART and SMARTER goals	Sometimes, things might not go so well because the goals were not SMART or SMARTER. Use this tool to check out the Specifics, Measurability, Agreed upon, Realistic, Time-based, Energising or Recorded.
Chapter 7	Template for leading a working/action group	This template could help you prepare for any difficult meetings that you might have to have with stakeholders when things are not good.
Chapter 8	Problem-solving tool (available on companion website)	This framework helps you to analyse your problem so that you can understand what is going on. This understanding leads to developing informed action plans.
	Evaluation and process review of group work and meetings	If it is your group work or meetings that are not going well, then you might find it helpful to find out why so that you can begin to put it right. Evaluating and reviewing the processes and the way people experience them might shed light on what you need to do to get things on the right track again.
	Giving and receiving feedback handout Indicators of effective feedback (available on companion website)	Giving and receiving feedback about things that are not so good is essential to move things on but it has to be done very sensitively and in a skilled way. These materials are worth looking at, before you have to do this, to remind yourself of the principles of giving feedback constructively to bring about positive change.
	Enabling questions	If you are helping an individual or group to explore what didn't go well, remember that enabling questions are more likely to help people, if appropriate, to own or share responsibility for it and to make action plans to redress it.

Activity 9.1: Acknowledging our own part in what didn't go well

This activity is for the care setting team, patients/residents and family members

This activity takes you back to the personal creative visualisation or thinking back to your experience of the practice development journey that you may have done in the bonus online chapter to acknowledge your part in the success of the practice development journey in the care setting. We encouraged you there to let anything that didn't go so well to float away. If something negative came up for you there, this activity gives you the opportunity to work with it now and think about how you can deal with any negative emotions that have come up and what you might do to redress them.

If you didn't do the visualisation activity on your achievements in the bonus online chapter (**www.wiley.com/go/ practicedevelopment/workbook**), we suggest that you do it before you do this one below that focuses on the difficulties. This order is important because focusing first on the negatives risks losing sight of the positives and achievements.

You will need:

- 20 minutes;
- your learning notebook;
- a quiet space in the workplace or its grounds to reflect on your own.

Key activities

Creative visualisation (5 mins) – after you have read these instructions, close your eyes. Tell yourself that you have 15 minutes learning space entirely for yourself.

Take a few deep breaths. Feel the rise and fall of your ribs. Hear the sound of your breath.

Remember your experience in the practice development as a river and acknowledge what you did/are achieve/achieving. Now, in your imagination, take yourself back to the source of the river (the starting point of the practice development). Make your way down the river again, experiencing all the difficulties in the twists and turns, the rocks and rapids, the waterfalls, quiet flows and pools. How do you see yourself, in your mind's eye, as you move down the river?

When you get to where you are now, gently open your eyes. Now reflect on the part you played and are playing now.

- What didn't go so well when you were navigating the difficult parts of your journey (the rocks, rapids, waterfalls, flows, pools)?
- What part did you play at those difficult points?
- If you are feeling emotional about what happened, think about whether you need support and how you would get it.
- If you feel you have something to learn or do, identify what, how and with whom. (10 mins)

Now make notes on what contribution you played to things not going so well and what you are going to do about it. You might decide, as an action, to look at the previous table to identify any materials in this pack that could be worth looking at. (5 mins)

What would you like to see yourself doing differently between now and the next time you review your contribution?

Activity 9.2: Helping each other learn from what didn't go well and work out what to do about it

This activity is for everyone in the care setting team

Do you find it difficult at work to share what you haven't done so well with co-workers, patients/residents and their families? Are you embarrassed to tell others or are you afraid that others might think you are useless at your job? Or is it just not done in the care setting, so you and everyone else never admit a part in something that didn't go well? Or maybe the culture in the care setting is still to put blame on a person or group rather than see a mistake or crisis (something going wrong or not as planned) as an opportunity for learning, growth and improvement.

Option 1: Working in threes (presenter, helper and observer)

The purpose of this first activity is to help you to begin to share those things with others and help them to share theirs. This activity can help you to develop the confidence to reveal perhaps some inadequacy or omission on your part, both to yourself and another person/group when they are helping you to learn from your practice and your mistakes. The activity also gives you a further chance to practise the enabling questions that we introduced you to in Chapter 8 and get more feedback on how you ask such questions and the effect they had. The activity can be done with your buddy, but preferably with three of you. It will take approximately 40 minutes with your buddy or 60 minutes in a three. It is best to do this activity with the people you do the achievements activity with in the bonus online Chapter (Activity 1, **www.wiley.com/go/practicedevelopment/workbook**) so that they also know what you did well and can use this knowledge to support you.

You will need:

- to have done Activity 1 in this chapter and Activity 1 in the bonus online chapter in advance. Therefore, you have written reflections on what you achieved, what was not so good and what you want to do about it in your learning notebook;
- a space to sit together somewhere private in the workplace or grounds;
- to check your ground rules;
- to negotiate with co-workers that you will not be interrupted.

Key activities

If you are only working with your buddy, you will be an observer at the same time as a presenter or helper. The timing for each presentation is 15 minutes including acknowledging anything painful or difficult in a supportive way by the helper and 5 minutes for feedback.

Presenter

You are to share something that you alone or with others have experienced as not going well in the practice development journey. You will discuss it with the helper. Try to be brief and specific. Although the whole event or story you describe might not be all negative, stick to the negatives that came out of it. (10 mins)

Helper

You are to help the presenter (within these 10 minutes) by trying to get the presenter to think through his or her part in what didn't go well and how it didn't. You could ask the observer to let you know when the 10 minutes are up. Ask open questions (How do you know? What does this mean?). The object is to help the presenter to define or redefine the achievement and their part in it in specific detail, so that the presenter can think about the impact of this achievement on her/him self, patients/residents and colleagues and what this might mean for the practice development. Some enabling questions that focus on the negative things that have happened may include:

- It sounds as though you are feeling . . .? Tell me more about it.
- What negative feelings do you have from this event . . .?
- How do you feel . . .?
- What do you think made it unsuccessful . . .?

- What sense do you have of how you might have contributed to the lack of success?
- How have you helped yourself to come to terms with any contribution you might have made?
- How can you learn from this?

After 10 minutes, the helper acknowledges and appreciates the presenter's feelings, honesty and desire to learn from this experience and move on. The helper gives detail of why s(he) thinks it wasn't successful too. The helper must not ask questions that focus on positive aspects of the event or story or unpick them, but reminds the presenter not to forget the achievements. The focus here is on seeing how the negative can be reframed as an opportunity for learning and for affirming plans to move things on. (5 mins)

Observer

The observer listens to what is being *said* (during the whole 15 minutes). You observe the verbal interaction (for example, is the presenter able to be positive about moving on?) and consider what questions/responses were more/less helpful in enabling the presenter to share and acknowledge his or her contribution to what didn't go well. Notice the impact of the acknowledgement and appreciation on the presenter. The observer also listens to/senses (with the body and imagination) what the *feelings* of the presenter and helper are in relation to moving on.

Finally, the observer also listens to /senses what the presenter has *invested* (or not) in reframing the negative to positive. What is the presenter's *will*, *commitment* or *motivation* toward building on / facing the negative to enhance the practice development?

Further points the observer may wish to consider include:

- Is the helper conveying the acknowledgement and appreciation in a way that feels real?
- What is the effect of the acknowledgement of what the presenter has gone through and affirmation of what they plan to do?
- Is the presenter focusing on the negative of what they have done and how to learn from it?

After the session and a pause, the presenter and helper (in that order) convey how the experience was for them (1 minute each). The observer then gives feedback for 5 minutes to the helper on how their facilitation helped the presenter, and also to the presenter. After that, the presenter and helper may wish to add their comments. Change roles, in order that each person in the two or three can take on the role of helper and presenter.

Option 2: After Action Review (AAR)

See the After Action Review Toolkit on the following pages that will help you set up and facilitate an AAR.

The After Action Review (AAR) Toolkit   For more information about AARs, google AAR, or try:

www.queri.research.va.gov/ciprs/projects/after_action_review.pdf
www.mildlydiverting.com/afteractionreview/index.shtml

What is an AAR?

The AAR is a simple process used by a team to capture the lessons learned from past successes and failures with the goal of improving future performance. It is an opportunity for a team to reflect on a project, activity, event or task so that the next time, they can do better.

Why would you conduct an AAR?

The AAR will not only make learning conscious within a team, but it can also help build trust amongst the team's members.

Who participates in an AAR?

Participants of an AAR should include all members of the team. A facilitator should be appointed to help create an open environment, promote discussion and draw out lessons learned.

When do you conduct an AAR?

AARs should be carried out immediately while the team is still available and memories are fresh. It is recommended that AARs should be incorporated at key points during a project, activity, event or task in the early planning stage though they are often completed at the end.

How long should an AAR take?

AARs can be powerful processes because of their simplicity. AARs can be conducted almost anywhere and will vary in length. For example, a 15 minute AAR can be conducted after a one-day workshop, or a much longer meeting could be held to reflect on the roll-out of a large-scale project.

How do you conduct an AAR?

Creating the right environment is critical. Participants unfamiliar with the AAR process should be given information on what it is all about and why it is being done. Particular emphasis should be made that AARs are used to promote learning and make it explicit, rather than on seeking out individuals to blame for past failures.

Asking the right questions: There are different ways to conduct AARs. Facilitators and groups are encouraged to experiment with the process and find the right questions that will work best with their group and the project, activity, event or task that is being reviewed. They should also attempt to keep the process as simple as possible. As a guideline, the following three sets of questions are suggested:

1. What was supposed to happen? What actually happened? Why were there differences?
2. What worked? What didn't? Why?
3. What would you do differently next time?

It is recommended that the facilitator posts the sets of questions on a flipchart or whiteboard to be briefly reviewed prior to seeking out the answers.

1. What was supposed to happen? What actually happened? Why were there differences?
   These questions are intended to create a shared understanding within the group on what were the initial objectives of the project, activity, event or task and whether they were achieved as planned. It is the role of the facilitator to encourage and promote discussion around these questions.
   Differences between reality and planned should be highlighted and insights into why there were differences should be further explored.
2. What worked? What didn't? Why?
   This set of questions focuses on generating conversation about what worked and didn't work during the course of the project, activity, event or task.
   First, the facilitator asks the team members what aspects of the project, activity, event or task worked for them. Additional probing questions could include 'What did they like?' or 'What are things that would be worthwhile repeating?' The facilitator should repeatedly follow up the team members' responses with the question 'Why?' to help generate a better understanding of the root causes of the successes.
   The facilitator then asks the team members what aspects of the project, activity, event or task didn't go so well or 'What were aspects that they didn't like?' Again, the facilitator should use the 'Why?' question to identify the root reasons or explanations as to why things didn't go so well.
   Tip: If suggestions are not forthcoming, the facilitator could go around the room asking each individual to express one thing that worked and one thing that didn't. Alternatively, if the participants have difficultly being open, you can also start with writing down comments on sticky notes and discussing them in the group afterwards.
3. What would you do differently next time?
   This question is intended to help identify Specific Actionable Recommendations (SARs). The facilitator asks the team members for crisp and clear, achievable and future-oriented recommendations.
   The facilitator should arrange in advance for an individual to capture the quotes connected to each SAR. They supplement the SAR and can be included in the documentation of the AAR.

The following provides an example of two ways to write up a SAR from an AAR conducted following the deployment of a new software application across an organisation:

🗵 **Poor SAR:** *More time to better understand the evidence.*

☑ **Better SAR:** *Complete evidence analysis by next week.*

Captured Quote: *'If we could get our hands on the training packs for use here we could provide better training' – Gillian*

Tip: The question could also be asked as 'If you could do this all over again, what would you do differently?'

Tip: Ask each individual to write down their response to the question 'What mark out of 10 would you give this project, activity, event or task?' Once everyone has written down their response, get each individual to tell the team their mark and then respond to the follow-up question 'What would make it a 10?'

The After Action Review (AAR) Toolkit

Capturing learning – An AAR template   Learning captured in an AAR can be documented and entered into a paper form or onto a searchable file format such as a database for later usage. The following template is provided as a guide. Once the document is complete, the facilitator must make sure that it is circulated to all AAR participants for their comments and feedback.

Name of Event:	
Date of Event:	
One or two sentences giving the background / scope of the experience:	
Sponsor – individual(s) who called the AAR:	
Key Particpants in the AAR	
AAR Facilitator:	
Key Words: (maximum of 10 that would enable future users to refind this learning)	

Specific Actionable Recommendations (SARs)	Quotes

Activity 9.3: Acknowledging, in the working day, when things don't go well and affirming plans to change

> This activity is for the clinical leader, team members and manager

Are you skilled in acknowledging others' experiences of things that don't go well? Do you give praise when people respond constructively by analysing what went wrong and developing plans to change themselves and/or their actions? Do you do these things informally in your working day when it is appropriate? Do you do them formally and intentionally in regular staff and patient/resident meetings and in practice development sessions? Especially if you are the team leader or manager, do you praise people's efforts to move things on in the corridor, public spaces, meetings, staff development reviews and personal development planning?

Are you able to recognise for yourself (when you have been offered feedback about something that didn't go so well) that the person feeding back is doing it intentionally to help you to reframe, learn and move things on? Often people aren't able to recognise this and so do not hear the affirmation of their attempts to reframe, learn and go forward. Thus they feel they are never offered recognition or praise for moving on when in fact they aren't able to see it for themselves.

The purpose of this solo activity is to help you to answer the questions posed in Activities 9.1 and 9.2 above and for you to recognise when you have received recognition and praise for your efforts to change yourself/actions.

Key activities

1. Keep a log in your learning notebook of when you acknowledge another person's recognition that they were part of something unsuccessful and affirm/praise their plans to turn it into something successful.
2. Reflect on the impact that giving such acknowledgement, affirmation and praise, where it is due, is having on the person, you and the practice development.
3. Note when you have received recognition and praise for your plans to change, improve and move on.

Good luck!

Remember to include patients/residents and family members in this too.
You could use the logbook template in the bonus online chapter or both your learning log and reflection.

Chapter 10　Practice Development as a Continuous Process

Introduction

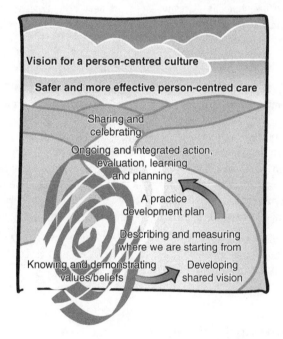

Fig. 10.1 Practice development as a continuous process

After many stops to pause on the way and celebrate the achievement of milestones on the journey to person-centred care, you and the care setting team have turned a corner. The practice development path still continues to stretch out in front of you!

As we have pointed out throughout this resource, practice development is a continuous way of working and being. Being and becoming a more effective practitioner in providing person-centred care of patients/residents never ends. It is not a project with a beginning and an end (even though your journey may look like a series of projects or several projects running together). The journey to becoming more person-centred and effective, and the learning, helping and evaluating that it takes, is always ongoing. This final chapter is designed for care setting teams to help them to keep motivated. Activities, guidance and examples are offered to help people pay attention to looking after themselves and keeping the practice development fresh. Linking to new policy agendas is aimed at the leaders, coordinators and facilitators of the practice development (including managers and executive teams).

Practice Development Workbook for Nursing, Health and Social Care Teams, First Edition. Jan Dewing, Brendan McCormack, and Angie Titchen.
© 2014 John Wiley & Sons, Ltd. Published 2014 by John Wiley & Sons, Ltd.
Companion website: www.wiley.com/go/practicedevelopment/workbook

In the bonus online chapter (**www.wiley.com/go/practicedevelopment/workbook**) we stress the importance of celebrating your successes, to motivate and energise you for the next steps on the journey. However, there is always a danger that you might become stuck or stagnant – and that you have to be aware of this danger. Otherwise, you might miss opportunities, for instance, to help a co-worker to become more person-centred or you may fall back into old, task-focused ways and deny a patient/resident a voice in making choices and decisions about their own care. Practice developers need to be constantly vigilant – watching their own practices and those of others to strive to live the person-centred vision.

We look at how you can keep your motivation and energy going by seeing each moment, day and week as a fresh opportunity to be creative, for example to get some idea across, to ask an enabling question or point out something that shows that a person-centred learning culture or infrastructure is beginning to happen or not.

We highlight that 'doing' practice development means that you are never really off the case! It's a bit like keeping lots of plates spinning at the same time. Because practice development is not easy and people are a mass of contradictions and resistances, everyone, but particularly those leading the changes, will need to attend to developments and people continuously. Even when we want to change, we can so often and easily slip back into, for example, using non-person-centred language or task-focused ways of working together and caring for patients/residents. Therefore, we offer suggestions for ways you can keep your practice development fresh and at the front of your heart and mind. We also look at how you can re-invent practice development to face new and unexpected challenges that arise and how, particularly, leaders can link practice development to new policy agendas for the best interests of patients/residents, families, teams and the organisation.

Resources in this chapter

1. **Look after yourself and your health** – an activity and links to information that remind you to care for yourself and your health
2. **Keeping it fresh everyday** – an activity and guidance to help you think through how you can keep practice development fresh when you find yourself and others becoming stale.
3. **The art of re-invention** – an example and activity to consider how to re-invent your practice development approach when new contextual and cultural challenges arise that make your approach unworkable.
4. **Linking to new policy agendas** – drawing on the policy agendas described in this resource, examples are used to show how practice development can be strengthened by linking it to these agendas. An activity is offered.

Activity 10.1: Look after yourself and your health

> This activity is for everyone in the care setting team

It's vital that you take care of your own health when caring for others. Being energised when you are at work will help you be focused on caring and probably improve your patience and stamina. Feeling tired, lethargic, run down, hungry and craving nicotine or sugar will reduce your ability to help others.

Ask yourself the following questions:

- What do I do to help my health?
- Can I do it better and if so, how?
- How healthy is my workplace?
- How can we make it healthier?

Change 4 Life Change 4 Life is a society-wide movement that aims to prevent people from becoming overweight by encouraging them to eat better and move more. The campaign aims to inspire a societal movement in which everyone who has an interest in preventing obesity, be they Government, business, health-care professionals, charities, schools, families or individuals, can play their part. (www.dh.gov.uk/en/Publichealth/Change4Life/index.htm)

Activity 10.2: Keeping it fresh everyday

This activity is for everyone in the care setting team

The purpose of this activity is to jump-start creativity when you find yourself and others becoming stale or falling into new ruts in your practice development. At times when you have stopped being mindful or active in your learning, doing, being and becoming, it will help you to draw on your own (and others') resources to devise ways of keeping your practice development fresh in your hearts and minds. Try to work with this guidance.

The activity can be done on your own, with your buddy or in a small, informal group (like an active learning group). You will need:

- approximately 30–45 mins;
- one of you to be facilitator if you are working in a group;
- ground rules (see Chapter 2);
- a space to move around in;
- your notebook;
- flipchart paper;
- materials, which could include felt-tip pens, paints, crayons, pastels, coloured paper or card (plus any other drawing materials you may want);
- a camera.

Key activities

This activity involves creating a short comic strip about transforming your practice development from staleness to freshness.

If you are facilitating a group activity, explain the purpose and key activities and structure the session. You can take part as well, but you will need to keep an eye on the timings.

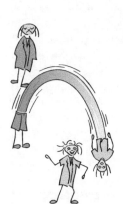

Walk around the space you are in, taking a few deep breaths. Pay attention to how you are holding your body and remember the body sensations you had at the start of the practice development journey. Remember those feelings you have felt as you have gone along the path . . . and finally, focus on the sensations of becoming stale (e.g. bored, uninspired, can't be bothered). (5 mins)

Sit down or continue standing or moving around if you want, and briefly note down or draw these sensations and when you felt them on the journey. (5 mins)

If you are with your buddy or group, share these sensations and point to the part of your body where you felt them. Help each other express the sensations. Use your bodies to do so. (5 mins with buddy or 10 mins with group)

Individually, each person then creates their own comic strip of three pictures, one representing your staleness, the next how to move to freshness and the third how you will feel when you come fresh to your practice development.

You can add speech bubbles to the characters and text to each of the cartoons. (10 mins)

If you are doing this activity with a buddy or a group, share your comic strips and ask each other enabling questions to help draw out insights and new ideas to help you keep your practice development fresh. (15 mins)

Record in your notebook the key thoughts and ideas for keeping the way you approach practice development fresh, and take a photo of your comic strips.

Postscript

After the activity, you might like to reflect further on instances when you recognise that you were slipping back into old, non-person-centred ways or language using one of the reflective tools in Chapter 4 and set up a session with your buddy to help you explore more deeply how you will act when you identify this happening again in your practice.

You might decide to share the comic strips with others in the care setting to stimulate discussion about what they mean and thus alert others to the importance of keeping things fresh.

Guidance: Keeping practice development fresh

> ### This activity is for everyone in the care setting team

Here are some ideas to help.

- Stay healthy.
- High challenge with high support is vital for keeping us fresh and constantly looking at ourselves and our practices – seek constructive feedback and seek support when you need it.
- Meeting regularly with your buddy or active learning group – learning with others is often much more fun as well as more challenging and energising than thinking things through on our own.
- Also meet as often as you can with your mini-project or practice development group to keep fresh ideas coming – use the activities in this resources at these sessions to explore whatever is problematic or relevant to the practice development at that time.
- Look out for learning networks set up in your area and make the effort to go along.
- Don't forget networking in your community, browsing the websites we have pointed out in this resource, and watching the videos to get a new take on things.
- Be alert to opportunities when you can hold up a 'mirror' for each other and reflect back to the other when things are going stale or unquestioned. This alertness keeps you fresh because you have to be creative to use what is happening in the here and now and tailor it for your purpose.

Example

A mini-project group working on improving multi-disciplinary care planning in a haematology unit has been struggling to make progress. Facilitated by Vera (the group lead and one of the nursing team leaders), group members have set up a conversation space for professional team members to explore, with patients and their family members, a person-centred planning framework for patient care. However, only a very few professional team members and no patients or families in the unit have shown any interest in attending. At one of their meetings, Vera suggests that the group should use the problem-solving tool in the companion website to understand the problem better. As usual, she leads and does most of the talking and decides what should be written in which box on the tool. When they get to the explanation of the problem, Sandy takes a deep breath and speaks up. 'It seems to me that the problem is that we haven't engaged everyone in setting up this project. We haven't involved patients or families or our colleagues sufficiently in setting up this project. And I think this stems from the fact that this is the way we work in this unit.' After a difficult pause, she goes on, 'What's more, we mirror that in this group. I say this, Vera, in recognition of all the energy you are putting into this group, but we (indicating with her hand, herself and other group members) let Vera do all the work and the talking and we don't challenge her or ourselves about this. We are passive and we prefer not to rock the boat and so we wait for Vera to tell us what to do. I'm bored with this now – we are becoming stale and I think we need to pay attention to creating a more person-centred culture in this group. Then I think we will be able to practise the skills for being collaborative, inclusive and participative with others in improving our person-centred care planning.'

There is silence for a while and Vera doesn't know what to say at first. Vera realises that Sandy is right – once again in her enthusiasm to get things done she has taken over. Although she feels upset and embarrassed, she decides to say 'Yes, you are right, Sandy, I am very sorry.' She pauses to think and then says 'I need the group to talk about this and for us to work together differently from now on.'

Examples: The art of re-invention

To help you understand by the art of re-invention in practice development, we give you three examples.

Examples of re-inventing practice development

1. A new senior manager is appointed with very different ideas about developing practice from the ones promoted in this resource. She wants to bring in an external consultant she has worked with in the past to 'sort out' the 'so-called' integrated care pathway for patients with diabetes. The practice development coordinating group is currently pulling together the baseline evaluation evidence that has been collected by nursing staff in the ward, the consultant nurse with a responsibility for patients with diabetes, the pharmacist and community nurses to create a practice development plan together. When they hear this news about the management consultant, they agree that they have to put the evaluation and planning on hold and act fast before the consultant is hired. The group redefine themselves, for now, as a lobby group to influence this senior manager's view. They develop a plan that starts with going to see the manager and sharing their work. As soon as the consultant is hired they arrange for the two of them to attend a mini-project team session working group session.

2. A new, blanket organisational policy about restricting staff and resident travel outside the care setting has been set in place by the organisation. This policy has upset a mini-project group's arrangements for meeting with community groups to discuss collaborations for enhancing the lives of patients/residents. Rather than just accept the situation and give up, they see that they must become more political to influence this decision. They decide to use national policy to help fight their case for these meetings to be given priority and for a limited travel budget to be negotiated for this important work. In the meantime others agree that meetings can be held in the care setting and the manager offers support for this to happen.

3. A new policy is being brought out on nutrition that requires your oncology ward to carry out an audit of MUST scores. A practice development project in your ward has been working on MUST and nutritional promotion/healthy eating for patients and you have baseline scores already carried out. However, you recorded these in a different way to the paper work that has been sent out. The group decides to remind the director of quality in the Trust that the scores have been done and that you have plans to repeat the measurement in 3 month's time after staff education has been completed. The director asks lots of questions and decides to speak with the audit project lead. She comes back and says that the baseline will be acceptable and that the audit lead was impressed with the work and would like to come and find out more about what is happening in your ward.

Activity 10.3: The art of re-invention

These three activities are suitable for everyone in the care setting team

The purpose of these activities is to help you to consider how you can reframe your development of practice or your approach to respond effectively to unexpected challenges that emerge in the context you are working in. There always will be challenges, so thinking quickly and creatively is necessary at these times.

Option 1: Reflection activity

This is a reflection activity that you can do on your own or with a colleague such as your buddy who poses the questions to you. The aim is to do this at a fairly quick pace – so that you say things quickly and don't dwell on them too much. Your buddy writes down the key words you say.

- What values and beliefs do you still hold that no longer serve your patients/residents well?
- What new values and beliefs do you need to adopt?
- What new beliefs or ideas do you need to put into action in order to improve your personal effectiveness?
- How can you put the new ideas and belief structures into action in your daily life?
- What will you read, study and learn that will help you become more person-centred?
- What will you stop spending your time and energy on?
- What three actions will you take to being more person-centred?
- What changes will others notice in you?
- What changes will others notice in your behaviours and your actions? Will the changes you make be enough for them to be visible to those around you? Are they significant enough to be noticed?
- How will these changes impact on patients/residents?

Option 2: The 're-invention game'

This game can be done with your buddy or small, informal group.
You will need:

- approximately 30 minutes;
- one of you to be facilitator if you are working in a group;
- ground rules (see Chapters 2 and 3);
- your notebook;
- felt-tip pens, coloured paper or card, safety pins.

Key activities

If you are facilitating a group activity, explain the purpose and key activities and structure the session. You can take part as well, but you will need to keep an eye on the timings.

Individually, think of an example of something unexpected that has happened in your workplace with the result that the practice development approach that has been adopted is no longer working. (1 min)

Ask yourself the following questions about it:

- What are the Strengths, Weaknesses, Opportunities and Threats (SWOT analysis in Chapter 5) in this new situation?
- How can you build on the strengths and opportunities and address the weaknesses and threats to re-invent or reframe the way you have been working as a practice developer? How can you think of yourself or selves differently and having a different function? (10 mins)

Choose one of your re-inventions and write it on a card without anyone seeing it.

Choose a partner and pin your card on her/his back with the safety pin (without them seeing what you have written on it) and vice versa. (2 mins)

You take turns to ask questions to find out what is written on your own back. Your partner can respond with words and/or mime. The winner is the person who finds out first. (10 mins, i.e. 5 mins each way)

If you are in a group, you then share the re-inventions with each other. (7 mins)

Option 3: Naming activity

Sometimes we need to rename the project we are doing so that it is more catchy or relevant to something that is going on in the organisation, locally or nationally. This can often help your project be more noticed and seem to fit better with broader policy or practice development.

This activity can be done by a small group of people or by putting up flipchart papers on the wall (you might call it a graffiti wall!) for a week and collecting in the responses. You can also make this into a small competition and award a small prize at the end.

Note: Consider the ways in which patients/residents and families can contribute to this activity.

Linking to new policy agendas

This final resource is aimed at those leading, coordinating or facilitating the development of practice in the care setting, including managers and executive managers

In this resource, we have hinted on occasion to the importance of linking your practice development plans and proposals to relevant health and social care policy agendas. Doing this strengthens your argument or case and key decision-makers in your care setting are more likely to sit up and take notice of what you are proposing. We showed you how this could work in the second example on the art of re-invention in the previous section. Your organisation's managers know that it will be judged by its implementation of national strategies and other agendas like QIPP (Quality, Innovation, Productivity, Prevention) and NHS Change (www.changemodel.nhs.uk/pg/dashboard). So if you can show the people who make strategic decisions in your organisation that your practice development proposal will help the organisation to do well, for example, in the next inspection by the Care Quality Commission, then you are more likely to get funding/support.

The way that policies are to be made in the future seems likely to change – yet again. Rather than being made at central government level, policies will be increasingly made at regional and even local level, which will affect you and which you and your organisation can influence through your practice development initiatives. There will always be new policies coming through to take into account.

The point of saying all of this is that it is vital for you and your organisation/workplace to link with new policy agendas, like the provision of work-based learning by partnerships between workplaces and higher education, for example the emerging foundation degrees (see useful websites in Chapter 8). By being aware of, and linking in with the new policies and initiatives arising from them, your care setting has a better chance of becoming a place with recognised excellence, which is good for patients/residents, families, teams and for business!

You don't need to stop what you are doing but rather look at how what you are already doing and what you are planning to do fits with the policy agenda or targets.

We offer you a few practical tips now to help you to keep abreast of developments that might be relevant to you, the care team and services you provide in your care setting.

- Someone in your workplace takes responsibility for say 3 months to scan for new national and local policies and initiatives that could be useful to the practice development and the workplace. This can be done by checking on the Department of Health and other websites listed in Chapter 1 and throughout this resource. This responsibility could be rotated to ease the workload and to enable more people to develop internet skills and to become more skilled in identifying when policy agendas could be linked into practice development activities.
- See that several of the team sign up for e-based regular alerts, newsletters prepared by national and your local government (County Council) and your organisation.
- Subscribe to a practice-based journal or a practice development website such as Foundation of Nursing Studies (www.fons.org/) or Campaign for Learning (www.campaignforlearning.org.uk).
- Bring in the relevant policy agendas into your conversations with stakeholders and in your practice development plan to support the case you are making.
- Encourage different team members to join local networks and make sure they feed back information and resources.
- Keep the noticeboards up-to-date and fresh.

If you work in a care home, as well as the above:

- see about becoming a clinical placement for nursing and therapy learners;
- keep a look out for free local lectures and seminars;
- offer space in the home for local relatives' and carers' groups to meet;
- set up and maintain relationships with local universities, research groups and other networks – this means opening up the home and inviting people in.

We have come to the end of this workbook now. We hope that it will guide, help and support you in your efforts to enhancing person-centred care in your team and wherever you work.

Have a good journey!

Useful websites and resources

For ease of use, you can also find these on **www.wiley.com/go/practicedevelopment/workbook**

1. **Practice development: collaborative working in social care**
   Guidance on collaborative working (www.scie.org.uk/publications/guides/guide34/background/whatis.asp)

2. **Connect in Care**
   The purpose of Connect in Care is to support learning and practice development across all settings in order to improve the quality and experience of care for older people in Scotland. This site gives you access to practice development projects in care settings. When you have accessed the site, write in 'practice development' in the website search box. (www.connect-in-care.net/practice-development-themes/accessing-health-and-healthcare/connect-in-care-projects/152-nhs-24-and-care-care settings)

3. **Integration, Collaboration and Empowerment – Practice Development for a New Context**
   Introduces a framework for practice development in Scotland. (www.nhshealthquality.org/nhsqis/files/ClinicalGovernance_PDUFramework_APR09.pdf)

4. England Centre for Practice Development Facebook group. This is a closed group. Please send an request to join.

References

Allan, K. (2001) *Communication and Consultation: Exploring Ways for Staff to Involve People with Dementia in Developing Services.* Joseph Rowntree Foundation. The Policy Press, Bristol. (www.jrf.org.uk/bookshop/eBooks/186134810X.pdf).

Bate, P. (1995) *Strategies for Cultural Change.* Butterworth-Heinemann, Oxford.

Binnie, A. & Titchen, A. (1999) *Freedom to Practise: The Development of Patient-Centred Nursing.* Butterworth Heinemann, Oxford.

Boomer, C. & McCormack, B. (2008) Creating the conditions for growth: Report on the Royal Hospitals and Belfast City Hospitals collaborative practice development programme. University of Ulster, Belfast. (See also http://onlinelibrary.wiley.com/doi/10.1111/j.1365-2834.2010.01143.x/abstract)

Department of Health (2013) Meeting needs and reducing distress: The prevention and management of clinically related challenging behaviour in NHS settings. London; DH.

Dewing, J. (2007) Participatory research: a method for process consent with persons who have dementia. *Dementia: The International Journal of Social Research & Practice,* **6** (1), 11–25.

Dewing, J. (2008a) Becoming and being active learners and creating active learning workplaces: the value of active learning. In: *International Practice Development in Nursing and Healthcare* (eds B. McCormack, K. Manley & V. Wilson), pp. 273–294. Blackwell, Oxford.

Dewing, J. (2008b) Process consent and research with older persons living with dementia. *Association of Research Ethics Journal,* **4** (2), 59–64.

Dewing, J. (2009a) Moments of movement: active learning and practice development. *Nurse Education in Practice,* **10** (1), 22–26.

Dewing, J. (2009b) *Process Consent Documentation.* University of Wollongong Uniting Care Ageing South Eastern Region.

Dewing, J. & Titchen, A. (2007) *Workplace Resources for Practice Development.* Royal College of Nursing, London.

Dewing, J., McCormack, B., Manning, M., McGuinness, M., McCormack, G. & Devlin R (2007) The Development of Person-Centred Practice in Nursing Across Two Older Peoples Services in Ireland. Final Report. Unpublished Report.

Dewing, J., Moore, S., Wilder, E., Lohrey, R., Hoogesteger, J., Sale, Z. & Winstanley, C. (2011) Outcomes from a pilot project on workplace culture observations: getting evaluation and outcomes on the agenda. *International Practice Development Journal,* **1** (1), article 3. (www.fons.org/library/journal/volume1-issue1/article3)

Drennan, D. (1992) *Transforming Company Culture.* McGraw-Hill, London.

Edvardsson, D., Fetherstonhaugh, D., Nay, R. & Gibson, S. (2010). Development and initial testing of the Person-centred Care Assessment Tool (PCAT). *International Psychogeriatrics,* **22**, 101–108.

Evans, K., Hodkinson, P., Rainbird, H. & Unwin, L. with Fuller, A., Hodkinson, H., Kersh, N., Munro, A. & Senker, P. (2006) *Improving Workplace Learning.* Routledge, London.

Fink L. D. (1999) Active Learning. (http://commons.trincoll.edu/ctl/files/2013/08/Week-3-Active-Learning.pdf).

Fowler, J., Fenton, G. & Riley, J. (2007) Using solution-focused techniques in clinical supervision. *Nursing Times,* **103** (22), 30–31.

Garbett, R. & McCormack, B. (2002) A concept analysis of practice development. *NT Research,* **7** (2), 87–100.

Goleman, D. (2004) *Emotional Intelligence: Why it Can Matter More Than IQ.* Bloomsbury, London.

Gribben, B. & Cochrane, C. (2006) Critical companionship: our learning journey. *Practice Development in Health Care,* **5** (1), 14–19.

Guba, E.G. & Lincoln, Y.S. (1989) *Fourth Generation Evaluation.* Sage, Newbury Park.

Harvey, G., Loftus-Hills, A., Rycroft-Malone, J., Titchen, A., Kitson, A., McCormack, B. & Seers, K. (2002) Getting evidence into practice: the role and function of facilitation. *Journal of Advanced Nursing,* **37** (6), 577–588.

Haynes, J. & Janes, N. (2011) Visioning with service users: tensions and opportunities for a new facilitator. *International Practice Development Journal,* **1** (1), 8. (www.fons.org/library/journal.aspx).

Health Service Executive (2010) *Enhancing Care for Older People – A Guide to Practice Development Processes to Support and Enhance Care in Residential Settings for Older People.* Health Service Executive West, Tullamore, Republic of Ireland. ISBN: 978-1-906218-35-5.

Heron, J. (1989) *The Facilitator's Handbook.* Kogan Page, London.

Heron, J. (2004) *The Complete Facilitator's Handbook.* Kogan Page, London.

Hunnisett, H. (2011) From fixer to facilitator: going round in circles promotes change! *International Practice Development Journal,* **1** (2), 9. (www.fons.org/library/journal.aspx).

Johns, C. (2000) Guided reflection. In: *Reflective Practice in Nursing: The Growth of The Professional Practitioner,* Second edition (eds A.M. Palmer, S. Burns & C. Bulman). Blackwell, Oxford.

Manley, K. (1992) Quality Assurance: The Pathway To Excellence In Nursing. In: *Nursing Care: The Challenge to Change* (eds G. Bryzinska & M. Jolley). Edward Arnold, London.

Manley, K., Titchen, A. & Hardy, S. (2009) Work based learning in the context of contemporary healthcare education and practice: a concept analysis. *Practice Development in Healthcare*, **8** (2), 87–127.

Manley, K., McCormack, B. & Wilson, V. (2009) *International Practice Development in Nursing and Healthcare*. Blackwell, Oxford.

Manley, K., Sanders, K., Cardiff, S. & Webster, J. (2011) Effective workplace culture: the attributes, enabling factors and consequences of a new concept. *International Practice Development Journal*, **1** (2), 1.

McCormack, B. & McCance, T. (2006) Development of a framework for person-centred nursing. *Journal of Advanced Nursing*, **56** (5), 1–8.

McCormack, B. & McCance, T. (2010) *Person-centred Nursing: Theory, Models and Methods*. Blackwell Publishing, Oxford.

McCormack, B., Dewing, J., Breslin, L., Tobin, C., Manning, M., Coyne-Nevin, A., Kennedy, K. & Peelo-Kilroe, L. (2010) The Implementation of a Model of Person-Centred Practice in Older Person Settings. Office of the Nursing Services Director, Health Services Executive, Dublin. (www.ulster.ac.uk).

McCormack, B., Manley, K. & Titchen, A. (2013) *Practice Development in Nursing and Healthcare*. Second edition. John Wiley & Sons, Ltd, Chicester.

McGill, I. & Beaty, L. (2001) *Action Learning*. Second edition. Kogan Page, London, pp. 105–106.

Mezirow, J. (1990) How critical reflection triggers transformative learning. In: *Fostering Critical Reflection in Adulthood* (ed. J. Mezirow), pp. 1–20. Jossey-Bass Publishers, San Francisco.

Murray, S., Magill, J. & Pinfold, M. (2012) Transforming culture in the critical care environment – the building block of the journey. *International Practice Development Journal*, **2** (1), 5. (www.fons.org/library/journal.aspx).

Pritchard, E. & Dewing, J. (2000) A multi-method evaluation of an independent dementia care service and its approach. *Aging and Mental Health*, **5** (1), 63–72.

Rogers, C. (1967) *On Becoming a Person: A Therapist's View of Psychotherapy*. Constable, London.

Rogers, C. (1983) *Freedom to Learn for the 80's*. Charles E. Merrill, London.

Rogers, C. & Freiberg, H. J. (1994) *Freedom to Learn*. Third edition. Macmillan/Merrill, New York.

Rolfe, G., Freshwater, D. & Jasper, M. (2001) *Critical Reflection for Nursing and the Helping Professions: A User's Guide*. Palgrove, Basingstoke.

Rycroft-Malone, J., Kitson A., Harvey G., McCormack B., Seers K., Titchen A. & Estabrooks C. (2002) Getting evidence into practice: ingredients for change. *Nursing Standard*, **16** (37), 38–43.

Titchen, A. (2003) Critical companionship: part 1. *Nursing Standard*, **18** (9), 33–40.

Warfield, C. & Manley, K. (1990) Developing a new philosophy in the NDU. *Nursing Standard*, **4** (41), 27–30.

Wellington, B. & Austin, A. (1996) Orientations to reflective practice. *Educational Research*, **38**, 307–316.

Index

Page numbers in *italics* denote figures.

Practice Development Workbook for Nursing, Health and Social Care Teams, First Edition. Jan Dewing, Brendan McCormack, and Angie Titchen.
© 2014 John Wiley & Sons, Ltd. Published 2014 by John Wiley & Sons, Ltd.
Companion website: www.wiley.com/go/practicedevelopment/workbook